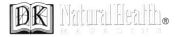

Secrets of

CHINESE HERBAL
MEDICINE

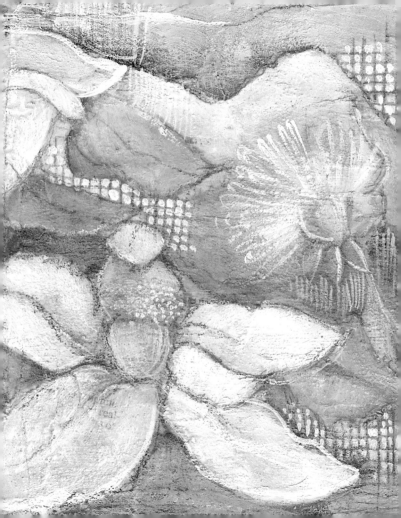

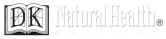

Secrets of

CHINESE HERBAL MEDICINE

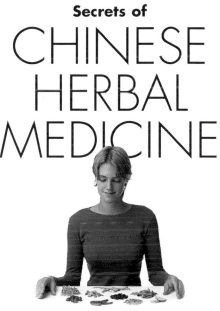

PENELOPE ODY

DK Publishing, Inc.

LONDON, NEW YORK, SYDNEY, DELHI, PARIS, MUNICH and JOHANNESBURG

This book was conceived, designed, and produced by
THE IVY PRESS LIMITED,
The Old Candlemakers,
Lewes, East Sussex DN7 2NZ

Art director Peter Bridgewater
Publisher Sophie Collins
Editorial director Steve Luck
Designers Kevin Knight, Jane Lanaway
Project editor Caroline Earle
Picture researchers Vanessa Fletcher, Trudi Valter
Photography Guy Ryecart
Illustrations Sarah Young, Nicola Evans, Andrew Kulman,
Pauline Allen, Ivan Hissey, Michael Courtney
Three-dimensional models Mark Jamieson

First published in The United States of America
in 2001 by
DK PUBLISHING, INC.,
95 Madison Avenue, New York, New York 10016

Natural Health ® is a registered trademark of Weider
Publications, Inc. Natural Health magazine is the leading
publication in the field of natural self-care. For subscription
information call 800–526–8440 or visit
www.naturalhealthmag.com

Copyright © 2001 The Ivy Press Limited

Note from the publisher
Information given in this book is not intended to be
taken as a replacement for medical advice. Any person
with a condition requiring medical attention should consult
a qualified medical practitioner or therapist.

A Cataloging in Publication record is available from the
Library of Congress

ISBN 0–7894–7776–9

Originated and printed by
Hong Kong Graphics and Printing Limited, China

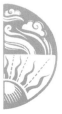

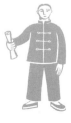

see our complete
catalog at

www.dk.com

CONTENTS

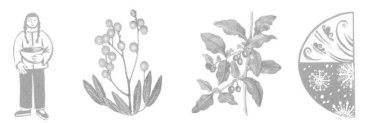

Chinese approach
Learn all about the Chinese herbal practitioner's approach to symptoms, diagnosis, and treatment.

HOW TO USE THIS BOOK
Secrets of Chinese Herbal Medicine is divided into two parts for ease of use. Part One outlines the history, theories, and principles behind Chinese herbal medicine, with information on consulting a practitioner and details of the types of remedies and how they are made. Part Two provides a comprehensive directory of herbs that may be prescribed by a practitioner, with pages listing the characteristics and action of each herb along with cautions on when not to use the remedy. The remedies in Part Two are grouped by function, such as herbs for clearing heat, warming the interior, clearing phlegm and dampness, and so on.

Important Notice

It is important to inform your doctor of any remedies or medications you are taking. Always observe the cautions, particularly if you are pregnant or have high blood pressure. Neither the author nor the publishers can be held responsible for claims arising from the inappropriate use of any remedy.

Do not use Chinese herbal remedies to replace medical treatment.

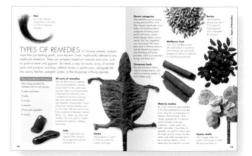

Background information
Historical facts and basic information on the Chinese remedies are given in Part One.

Practical

Full-color pages provide practical information with step-by-step photographs.

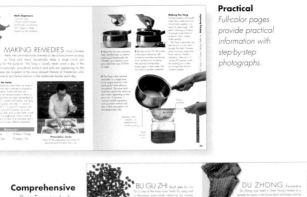

Comprehensive

Part Two includes comprehensive information on each remedy, including each herb's characteristics, dosage, actions, and contraindications.

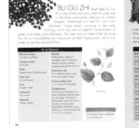

Detail

Black-and-white spreads give detailed information on each category of herbs.

Traditional Chinese Medicine

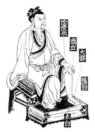

Ancient tradition
Chinese medical theories date back at least 5,000 years—TCM encompasses a variety of therapies.

Traditional Chinese Medicine (TCM) comprises an ancient group of therapies that have been practiced in China for at least 5,000 years. TCM combines techniques like acupuncture, massage, and moxabustion (burning herbs on acupuncture needles) with the use of plant, animal, and mineral remedies; dietary guidelines; and exercise routines that can be used for self-help. Like other traditional healing systems, TCM can appear obscure and exotic, having an alien vocabulary and concepts that can seem confusing.

TCM and the West

Over the past 30 years, forms of TCM have become more familiar and fashionable in the West: acupuncture is now acknowledged and used by many modern physicians while QiGong and t'ai chi exercise classes are widely available. Retail outlets for Chinese herbs, too, are now found in most large towns and cities, but support for these products remains mixed. Many remedies have received adverse publicity: some are derived from endangered species or involve the cruel treatment of animals, while others have been found to contain highly toxic chemicals. The quality of herbal remedies in some countries can also be suspect and, as a result, many professional therapists prefer to use products originating from Singapore, Japan, or California.

As with other alternative therapies that have become fashionable in the West, there has been an attempt at regulation by modern agencies and the use of many Chinese herbs is now restricted in Australia and some European countries.

This deters would-be patients from seeking help and adds to the general misunderstanding of what are often highly specialized and skilled treatments.

The Chinese herbal repertoire contains many plants that are familiar in the West either from their use in Western herbal medicine (such as dandelion and ginger), or as plants that we know only as garden ornamentals (like magnolia or forsythia). Many of these remedies have been well researched in the East, although Western studies can be limited, and have proven effective for a wide range of complaints. Some herbs are used in similar ways to their European relatives, but the traditional Chinese terminology describing their actions can be confusing. In the same way as Western herbal medicine, TCM is mainly concerned with helping the body to combat any imbalance and disharmony upsetting healthy equilibrium, rather than focusing on obliterating symptoms, as is the approach in modern allopathic medicine.

5,000 YEARS OF CHINESE
HERBAL MEDICINE

Humans have been using herbs to cure their ills since ancient times. For example, traces of Ma Huang (ephedra)—a Chinese herb used in asthma treatments and the source of our modern drug ephedrine—have been found in Iraqi tombs dating back 60,000 years. ✒ Chinese tradition dates the use of herbal remedies back to around 3000BC. The "Divine Farmer," Shen Nong, is credited with both tasting hundreds of herbs to identify their therapeutic properties and teaching the early Chinese the basics of agriculture and husbandry. ✒ His great herbal text, the *Shen Nong Ben Cao Jiang*, lists 365 medicinal products including herbs, minerals, and animals products. Today these same remedies still form the basis of many Chinese prescriptions that have continued in an almost unbroken tradition for at least 5,000 years.

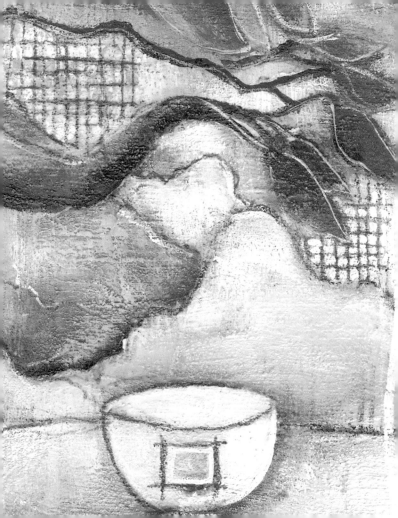

Shen Nong and the Yellow Emperor

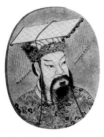

The Yellow Emperor
Huang Di is credited with much of TCM theory, although he is also the reputed founder of Chinese musical theories.

Chinese tradition credits Shen Nong with the discovery of medicinal herbs. His near contemporary, Huang Di or the Yellow Emperor, is believed to have formulated the basic theories of Chinese medicine. These survive in another of the great Chinese classics, the *Huang Di Nei Jing Su Wen* or *Yellow Emperor's Canon of Internal Medicine*, dated to c. 2500BC, although surviving manuscripts are c. 200AD.

As in the West, where medical practitioners were often priests or shamans, early Chinese medicine was also closely linked with religion—in this case Taoism. This ancient philosophy concentrates on achieving prosperity, longevity, and even immortality through "virtue"—which, to its followers, means conformity to nature both within the individual and beyond. Herbs, especially potent tonics like Ling Zhi (*Ganoderma lucidum*, a type of fungus), were regarded as being able to strengthen this adherence to virtue.

The Taoists based their beliefs on the world they saw around them—a world where the changing seasons gave rise to a model of five basic elements reflecting the growth and decline of vegetation. This also led to the belief in the dual nature of all things, which developed into the concepts of yin and yang as two equal but opposite primeval forces: beauty only exists because there is ugliness, light because of dark, male–female, hot–cold, and so on. The need to achieve balance between yin and yang, which was an important consideration for the Yellow Emperor, remains a core concept in Chinese medicine even today.

Complementary techniques

The *Yellow Emperor's Canon* was also the first to describe the various therapeutic techniques used in Chinese medicine that complement the herbal remedies of Shen Nong. These include acupuncture, massage, exercise therapies, moxabustion, and "plum blossom" treatments, which involve tapping specific points on the body with a tiny hammer set that incorporates nine needles.

More Information

For more information see Types of Remedies, pages 14–15; The Five Element Model, pages 38–39; Yin and Yang, pages 60–61; QiGong, pages 92–93.

Hair
Xu Yu Tan (charred human hair) is still used in TCM for bleeding disorders.

TYPES OF REMEDIES
A Chinese remedy contains more than just healing plants, since the term "herb" traditionally referred to any medicinal substance. There are remedies based on minerals and rocks, such as pumice stone and gypsum. But there is also an exotic array of animal parts and products including cuttlefish bones or earthworms, alongside the less savory leeches, pangolin scales, or the droppings of flying squirrels.

The Six Main Groups

Shen Nong classified his remedies into six main groups:

- jades and stones
- herbs
- woods
- animals
- fruits and vegetables
- cereals

All sorts of remedies
Xiao Shi (the mineral mirabilite), was recommended for clearing excess heat from the system and was also seen as a strong laxative. Chippings from stalactites were considered to be more warming and were used to treat frostbite and dysentery. Among Shen Nong's more exotic animal remedies was Liu Chu Mao—the hair and hooves from six species of domestic animals (horse, cow, sheep, pig, dog, and chicken). This was used to combat possession by demons, epilepsy, and mania.

Jade
Yu Xue (jade dust) was used by Shen Nong to encourage tissue growth and boost Qi.

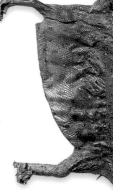

Gecko
Ge Jie (gecko) is used in TCM as a tonic for kidneys and lungs.

Eleven categories

Later herbalists such as Su Jing, writing around 659AD, took Shen Nong's classification even further. He produced eleven categories of healing plants: jewels and stones, weeds, human beings, beasts, poultry, insects, fish, fruit, vegetables, rice, and wood. The human parts used in Chinese medicine include charred hair (used to stop bleeding) and human placenta, which is an important energy and blood tonic.

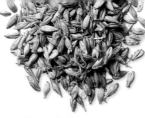

Barley

Mai Ya (barley sprouts) are used in TCM today for food stagnation and to strengthen the stomach.

Wolfberry fruit

Gou Qi Zi (wolfberry fruits) are used today for nourishing and tonifying liver and kidney energies as well as for deficient yin and blood syndromes.

Cinnamon bark

Rou Gui (cinnamon bark) is used to combat exterior cold and is a warming remedy to tonify kidney yang.

Materia medica

By 1590, when the great herbalist Li Shi Zhen published his book *Ben Cao Gang Mu*, (Compendium of Materia Medica) listed 1,892 "drugs" grouped into 16 sections which included "cloth and containers," scales, gold, fires, earth, and shells. Clam shells, for example, are used for certain types of coughs and for urinary disorders while oyster shells are believed to be a calming sedative, which means they are useful for insomnia.

Oyster shells

Mu Li (oyster shells) are used in TCM today to settle the spirit and help yin.

Characteristics of Herbs

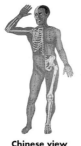

Chinese view

Traditional Chinese views of the body, and of plants and their properties, are different from the Western perspective.

Chinese herbal remedies are also classified, as they are in traditional Western medicine, by their intrinsic characteristics and the action they will have on the body.

In the days before chemical analysis it was impossible to classify remedies by the actions of their various constituents—such as the alkaloids, saponins, and steroidal compounds to which modern science now attributes their properties. Instead plants were defined by their temperature, taste, and the particular organs they were likely to affect. They were also defined in terms of the acupuncture channels that the herbs affected as well as, occasionally, by the directional influence they have once inside the body. An herb is described as:

• hot, warm, neutral, cool, or cold;

• sweet, sour, bitter, pungent, salty, astringent, or bland/neutral;

• entering the liver, lung, heart, kidney, spleen, gallbladder, large intestine, small intestine, urinary bladder, stomach, pericardium, or San Jiao (triple burner) meridians.

They are also sometimes described as lifting, lowering, floating, or sinking.

Applying the properties

As with the traditional forms of medicine practiced in Europe until well into the seventeenth century, Chinese herbs are used to counter-balance the symptoms of a disease and to restore order. Cold conditions, such as a chill or rheumatic aches and pains, are treated by warming herbs, while a fever or illness that involves heat is treated with cold herbs.

Chi Shao Yao (red peony root—see page 110) is classified as slightly cold with a sour and bitter taste affecting the liver meridian. It is a specific remedy for cooling problems that are associated with heat in the blood and so clears "liver fire." In Chinese theory the liver is associated with menstrual problems so Chi Shao Yao is given for period pains. Heat in the blood can also be linked to irritant skin rashes so it is sometimes included in prescriptions for eczema. It was actually one of the herbs that was used in the well-known trial using Chinese remedies for children suffering from severe eczema at Great Ormond Street Hospital, London, in the early 1990s (see pages 128–129).

Huang Qin (baical skullcap—see page 135) is classified as a cold herb and is used to treat a range of disorders involving heat or characterized by fever. Shan Yao (Chinese yam) is a neutral remedy that is not specifically hot or cold so it is suitable for a wider range of conditions.

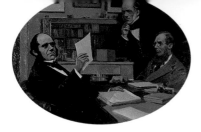

Joseph Dalton Hooker
During the 18th and 19th centuries Europeans like Sir Joseph Dalton Hooker traveled to China to seek out new plants for Western gardens.

THE PLANT HUNTERS
Although many of the plant species used in Chinese medicine seem strange and exotic to Westerners, others are also surprisingly familiar—not as medicinal herbs but as common garden shrubs. These were introduced into Europe beginning in the eighteenth century by the great plant hunters such as Robert Fortune, Sir Joseph Dalton Hooker, and Ernest Wilson who traveled extensively in China and Tibet. Plants were brought back to grace botanical gardens and private collections Their therapeutic properties, however, were ignored by Western botanists.

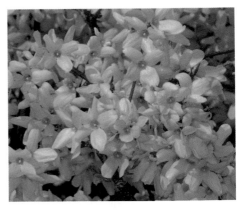

Forsythia
Lian Qiao (yellow-flowered forsythia fruits) are an important cooling remedy for clearing heat and toxins. The bush was introduced into Europe by Robert Fortune in 1844 who brought back tiny seedlings in specially made glass cases that were carried deep in the hold of his ship.

Magnolia

Several species of magnolia are used in Chinese medicine, although some varieties were not introduced into the West until the 1900s by the explorer Ernest Wilson. Xin Yi Hua (flowers of *Magnolia. liliiflora*) is used in China for colds and nasal mucus, while Hou Po and Hou Po Hua (bark and flowers of *Magnolia officinalis* respectively) help to stimulate digestive energies and ease abdominal distention.

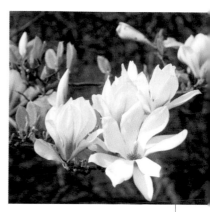

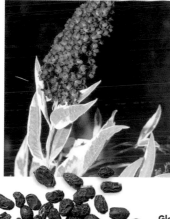

Buddleia

Purple-flowered buddleia bushes are almost a weed in many parts of Europe and are a familiar sight along London's railroad lines and embankments. Mi Meng Hua (buddleia flowers) is used in China for eye problems including conjunctivitis and cataracts.

Glossy privet fruits

Chinese privet was first brought to England by Sir Joseph Banks in 1794 and is now grown in Southern areas although it is not fully hardy. Nu Zhen Zi (glossy privet fruits) is an important tonic remedy for the liver and kidneys and the herb reputedly helps to darken graying hair as well as strengthen the knees.

Fighting the Weeds

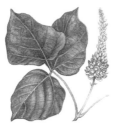

Kudzu vine
Introduced into North America in the 19th century as a fodder crop, kudzu is now a serious vegetative menace.

Not all the medicinal plants that have been introduced from China have proved quite so friendly in the West. A few, taken from their own balanced habitats, have become invasive weeds.

Among those in the "nuisance" category are Japanese honeysuckle from which the remedy Jin Yin Hua is made. A particularly virulent variety of this normally pleasant garden climber was developed in the 1860s at a New York nursery by George Hall. The plant soon escaped the garden and has become naturalized in many parts of the US as a virulent weed.

Perilla (*Perilla frutescens*)—a popular herb in Chinese cooking—has also become naturalized as a weed in many parts of the world. In China the seeds (Zi Su Zi), leaves (Zi Su Ye), and stems (Zi Su Geng) are used to treat colds, nasal mucus, and coughs. The leaves are often used in cooking—traditionally combined with crab so that the warming nature of the plant helps to balance the cold character of the shellfish.

Coping with kudzu

One of the most pernicious weeds, kudzu vine (*Pueraria lobata*), has been described as a "vegetative plague" in many southern US states. The herb, a member of the pea family, was introduced into the US from Japan in the 1870s and was welcomed as a potential food, fodder, and fiber crop. From 1910 to the early 1950s the planting of it was actively encouraged. By 1945 at least 500,000 acres in several southeastern states had been planted with the vines. Inevitably it self-seeded and spread unchecked across vast areas of arable farmland and proved very difficult to eradicate.

The many medicinal attributes of kudzu now seem forgotten in the huge effort there has been to eradicate the plant. In China, Ge Gen (kudzu root) and Ge Hua (kudzu flowers) are used medicinally. The root is used to encourage sweating in feverish colds and to relieve measles and neck pains, while studies have also shown it to be helpful for reducing high blood pressure and in the treatment of angina pectoris. The flowers are used in a traditional remedy to relieve alcohol poisoning and modern studies suggest that the whole plant can help reduce addiction to both drugs and alcohol.

More Information

For more information see **Ge Gen,** page 59; **Jin Yin Hua,** page 142; **Lian Qiao,** page 43; **Mi Meng Hua,** page 127; **Nu Zhen Zi,** page 79.

Herb dispensers

In ancient times, Chinese itinerant herbal practitioners would travel from village to village dispensing their remedies

MAKING REMEDIES

Most Chinese medicines are traditionally brewed as decoctions known as soup or Tang and many households keep a large crock pot specifically for the purpose. The Tang is usually taken once a day in the morning. Increasingly, powdered extracts and pills are appearing on the market. These are targeted at the more stressed lifestyle of Westerners who have little time to boil herbal extracts in the traditional manner each day.

Dispensing the herbs

In a Chinese dispensary dried herbs are stored in individual drawers and combined as required to make a prescription. Traditionally they are weighed on the old measures based on the Jin or caddy-full. These have now been standardized so a Jin equals 10½ ounces (300 grams), one Liang is 1 ounce (30 grams), one Qian ⅒ ounce (3 grams), one Fen is ¹⁄₁₀₀ ounce (0.3 grams), and one Li is ¹⁄₁₀₀₀ ounce (0.03 grams). Up to one Liang of a heavy herb, such as clam shells, would be prescribed in a single dose. More commonly there would be 3–5 Qian of an individual herb in a formula of four to twelve different ingredients.

Measures	
10 Li = 1 Fen	10 Qian = 1 Liang
10 Fen = 1 Qian	10 Liang = 1 Jin

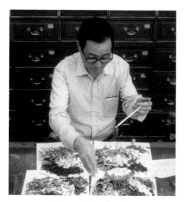

Prescription herbs

Herbs for the prescription are made into separate packs for each day's use.

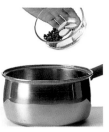 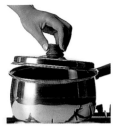

Making the Tang

Chinese patients will usually collect their medicines from a local herb supplier in a series of paper bags, with each containing a mixture of enough crude herbs to produce a day's supply of the remedy.

The Tang is generally very dark brown in color and strongly flavored. Chinese doses are much larger than those used by Western herbalists—often up to 3 ounces (90 grams) and the resulting mix is often too strongly flavored for Western palates.

1 Place the mix into a stainless steel, earthenware, or ceramic cooking pot (traditionally the Chinese use a ceramic crock pot). Add three cups (750ml) of water.

2 Boil the mix for 25–30 minutes so the liquid reduces by half. Sometimes remedies are brewed twice: boiled once, as above, then strained and the herbs boiled again in fresh water. The two extracts are then combined.

3 The Tang is then strained and taken In a single dose on an empty stomach in the morning (for more effective absorption). The same herbs might be used for the following day's brew depending on the exact mix If, however, it contains soluble ingredients, such as certain mineral salts, then a fresh prescription will be needed each day.

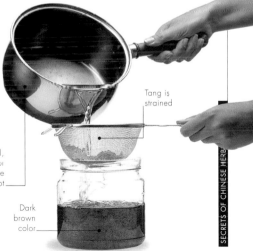

Tang is strained

Stainless steel, ceramic, or earthenware cooking pot

Dark brown color

All Sorts of Remedies

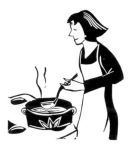

The Tang
Tangs are brewed in a traditional crock pot in Chinese households.

As well as decoctions or soups (Tang), Chinese herbs are also prescribed as powders (San) and pills (Wan). These are often more convenient to take since the remedy simply needs to be measured out each day rather than brewed. The dose of a powdered mixture is generally stirred into half a cup (125ml) of warm water while pills are traditionally made from ground herbs blended with honey and rolled into pellets. Many of the Tang mixtures are now also sold ready made as powdered extracts.

Although there is little difference between the powdered and crude herbs, some traditional Chinese practitioners believe that changing the style of the formulation could affect its therapeutics. Chinese herbs are also made into Western-style tinctures, which are made using alcohol and water. Alcohol itself is used in TCM as a warming therapeutic ingredient so tinctures may be more warming than the original herbal extracts. This could make a cooling remedy that is used to treat a hot condition less beneficial.

Making tonic wines

Tonic wines (Jiu) were popular with the ancient Taoists and are still made in China today. According to one legend, the sage Li Ch'ing Yuen died in 1930 at the age of 252 years. His long life was helped by a small glass of mixed He Shou Wu (flowery knotweed) and Ren Shen (Korean ginseng) tonic wine taken each evening before bed. Tonic wines are easy to make at home using a large vinegar vat filled with the tonic herb—

usually a root such as Dang Gui (Chinese angelica), He Shou Wu, or Ren Shen—which is then covered with red wine. The mix is left for a few weeks; up to 2½ fluid ounces (75ml) of the mixture can be drawn off for a daily dose. More wine should be added to prevent the damp herb from turning moldy.

Extracts can also be made using vodka or brandy to create therapeutic aperitifs or after-dinner liqueurs. Hu Tao Ren (walnuts) steeped in vodka for a month can be used as an energizing tonic drink for the kidneys, while Hong Zao (Chinese red dates) soaked in brandy for a month will produce a sweet-tasting liqueur that is good for the liver and blood.

More Information

Tonic wines can also be made using:

Bai Shao Yao, see page 110; **Bai Zhu**, see page 94; **Chen Pi**, see page 82; **Dan Shen**, see page 106; **Dang Shen**, see page 107; **Gan Jiang**, see page 146; **Huang Qi**, see page 91; **Wu Wei Zhi**, see page 203; **Xi Yang Shen**, see page 74; or **Xiao Hui Xiang**, see page 151.

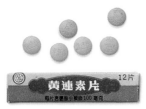

Pills

Many traditional prescriptions are now made into pills that are available as over-the-counter remedies.

黄連素片

12片

PRESCRIPTIONS

Herbal medicines in the West are often used individually or dispensed in various combinations that have been selected by the practitioner as appropriate to the particular patient and ailment. In China dispensing is far more structured, with thousands of detailed prescriptions matched to particular disease syndromes. These prescriptions may be adjusted slightly by physicians but are more often dispensed using a standard formula. These combinations are also used as standard in ready-made pills and powders that are available over-the-counter.

Herbal Formulas

Many traditional formulas have been used for centuries: the *Zheng Lei Ben Cao* written by Tang Shen-Wei in 1082 lists 300 classic "recipes" while Li Shi Zhen, writing in 1590, gives details of 11,096 individual prescriptions. Chinese medical students must learn many thousands of these formulas by heart during their training.

Within the prescription particular herbs fulfill precisely defined roles:

 Emperor the principal therapeutic herbs, such as Ren Shen (Korean ginseng) and Shu Di Huang (Chinese foxglove).

 Messenger included in some remedies to "target" the prescription to particular meridians or parts of the body.

 Minister herbs that support and strengthen the key plants, such as Bai Zhu (white atractylodes) and Dang Gui (Chinese angelica).

 Helper or Harmonizer auxiliary and/or correcting herbs that can counter any toxic effects within the major ingredients or treat secondary symptoms in the condition.

Herb Key

1. Ren Shen
2. Shu Di Huang
3. Bai Zhu
4. Dang Gui
5. Bai Shao Yao
6. Gan Cao
7. Sheng Jiang
8. Da Zao

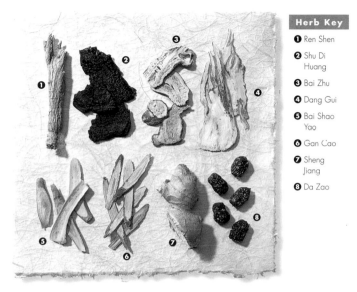

Women's precious pills

A typical traditional formula is Bu Zhen Tang —the eight ingredient decoction that is often marketed as "women's precious pills." This remedy is designed as an energy and blood tonic, and it contains the following herbs:

• Ren Shen (Korean ginseng) and Shu Di Huang (Chinese foxglove), the key *Emperor* herbs— potent tonics for energy and blood.

• Bai Zhu (white atractylodes), Dang Gui (Chinese angelica), and Bai Shao Yao (white peony), also effective tonics in the *Minister* role.

• Chuan Xiong (Sichuan lovage) and Fu Ling (tuckahoe) act as *Messenger* herbs to target the remedy.

• Gan Cao (licorice root), Sheng Jiang (fresh ginger), and Da Zao (Chinese dates) act as *Helper* herbs to balance its conflicting attributes.

Tonic

Women's precious pills are used in TCM for gynecological problems associated with energy or blood deficiency.

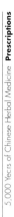

TCM Today

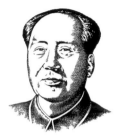

Mao Tse Tung
Under Mao Tse Tung, traditional remedies were revived with the establishment of new colleges devoted to the study of TCM.

Although Traditional Chinese Medicine continued to dominate China until the end of the eighteenth century, Western missionaries and anatomical science began to erode it. The first Chinese doctor to study in the West, Huang Kuan arrived at Edinburgh University in the 1860s. By the 1890s there was a College of Western Medicine in Hong Kong. By the time that the first Chinese Republic was established in 1911, government ministers were trying to suppress traditional medicine.

Emigrant Chinese in Singapore, California, Hong Kong, and "Chinatowns" around the world kept many of the old traditions alive. However, by the mid-twentieth century TCM in China itself survived as little more than folklore and household remedies.

The communist revolution

In 1949 traditional China changed forever when the communists under Mao Tse Tung seized power and decided that improving public health was a key priority. A major conference held a year later recommended combining Western teaching with a revival in China's traditional healing arts.

New colleges of Traditional Chinese Medicine were established and, by 1966, Mao's famous "barefoot doctors"—paramedics with basic training in traditional skills—were at work in remote country areas as the Chinese government battled to improve the poor levels of health and hygiene prevalent in many parts of China. The old remedies were reintroduced and new pharmaceutical plants were established in order to produce mass-market remedies for over-the-counter sale.

Although some of the tradition was lost during the Cultural Revolution in the 1970s, by the mid-1980s Western students were starting to study at the new colleges of TCM. As China adopted more open policies, a slow trickle of traditionally trained Chinese practitioners began to move West and join the small numbers of TCM doctors among emigrant Chinese communities.

Growing popularity

Over the past decade Chinese herbal remedies and formulas have become readily available in the West, and growing interest in Chinese medical theories has encouraged traditional practitioners to set up outlets. Today most reasonably sized towns will boast at least one Chinese herbal store with a resident physician. Remedies based on the ancient formulas are also now available in many conventional pharmacies and health food stores.

Pulse-taking
*In TCM the patient rests
each wrist in turn on a
small cushion so that the
practitioner can take a pulse
reading from them both.*

CONSULTING A PRACTITIONER

For modern Westerners, consulting a Chinese physician may at first seem very strange and exotic. The technique and approach, however, would be very familiar to a traditional eighteenth-century Western doctor since its emphasis is on close examination of the patient's appearance as well as incorporating thoughtful interrogation to identify symptoms and underlying causes of ill health.

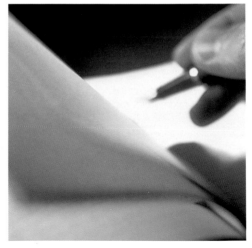

The consultation
A consultation with a TCM practitioner generally follows a well-established routine. The four stages of the consultation enable the practitioner to build up a detailed diagnosis. Once the examination is complete the practitioner will make a diagnosis, identifying the underlying syndrome, and will then prescribe herbs that the patient collects from the dispensary when leaving the clinic.

Looking

The practitioner starts by "looking"— examining the patient's appearance, facial expression, skin color, gait, demeanor, and general appearance. All these provide clues as to the underlying energy levels and vigor. A skilled physician takes in all he or she needs to know with a simple glance.

Hearing and smelling

This is followed by the "hearing and smelling" stage, which includes listening to the patient's voice and breathing rhythms as well as smelling any body odors. In the past "taste" was added to this stage in the diagnosis and physicians would taste their patient's urine to identify any sweetness, which could imply diabetes.

Questions and answers

Next the practitioner asks questions about particular symptoms as well as more general discussion on whether the patient feels hot or cold, thirsty or hungry, calm or restless, or whether there is any pain.

Touching

Finally comes palpation or touching, which focuses on pulse-taking. The physician will feel each wrist in turn for the nine basic pulses that help to guide diagnosis. The practitioner may also feel the body surface to assess temperature and quality and will check the nature of any swellings.

Modern TCM practitioners may also include the sort of clinical tests familiar in the West, such as taking a blood pressure reading or sending blood samples for analysis. However, these traditional four stages are still the basis of examination.

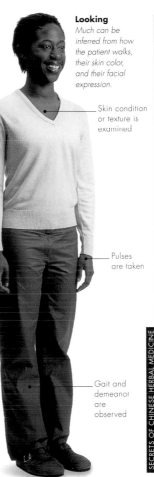

Looking

Much can be inferred from how the patient walks, their skin color, and their facial expression.

Skin condition or texture is examined

Pulses are taken

Gait and demeanor are observed

Controversial Chinese Remedies

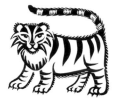

Endangered species
Wide use of tiger bones for joint pains is threatening rare species with extinction.

Chinese medicine has always used herbs, minerals, and animal parts in its remedies. Although some of them are offensive to Westerners, they continue to be popular. Production can often involve quite horrific treatment of endangered species and intensive "farming" of wild animals. The more unpleasant remedies are:

Hu Gu (tiger bones)—used for painful joint conditions;

Hai Ma (seahorses)—used as a kidney tonic, especially in the elderly suffering from general debility;

Hai Gou She (seal testes)—used to strengthen reproductive energy;

Xiong Dan (bear's gallbladder)—used to clear heat and toxins and reduce pain and swelling in sprains and fractures. None of these should be used today as there are many suitable alternatives.

Poor qualities

Many factories in mainland China also sell very dubious herbal remedies for export. These may be polluted with synthetic chemicals or contain plants that have little to do with the herbs they purportedly contain. These products can be toxic.

Confused names

The situation is not helped by a general confusion over Chinese plant names. Although they originate in different regions, different species are sometimes given the same Mandarin name because they are used in the same way. Fang Ji is usually *Stephania tetranda* but it can also mean *Cocculus trilocus* or *Aristolochia fangchi* in certain regions: all three herbs can be used as a diuretic (to stimulate urine flow) and painkiller. However, *Aristolochia spp.* are toxic and misuse can lead to kidney failure. A patent remedy sold in Belgium in the early 1990s as a diet aid was blamed for 70 cases of kidney failure as *Aristolochia fangchi* was used instead of the more usual *Stephania tetranda*. The result has been restrictions in many parts of Europe on anything labeled Mu Tong (chocolate vine) or Fang Ji. This confusion has done little to reassure patients and practitioners of the safety or efficacy of Chinese medicine.

Suppliers

Given the dubious quality of many Chinese herbal products, a number of practitioners prefer to use ready-made remedies produced in Japan, California, or Singapore. Crude herbs can be of doubtful origin so it is best to buy from a reputable mail-order supplier who can authenticate the source.

CHINESE
HERBAL REMEDIES

The traditional way of describing the actions of Chinese herbs can sound very confusing to Westerners. A plant may be described as "combating fire poisons," "draining damp," or "invigorating spleen energy." This reflects the way TCM regards illness as caused either by some sort of external "evil" or internal imbalance. ⟡ Herbal remedies are also grouped by exotic-sounding attributes so that while some traditional Chinese herbals will list remedies alphabetically, others classify remedies into subgroups such as "releasing exterior conditions," "regulating blood," or "clearing heat." ⟡ The herbs will almost always be used in complex formulas of at least three or four different remedies so the same herb can appear to have different properties.

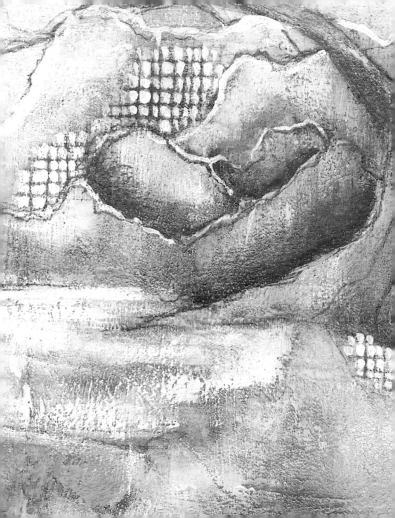

Chinese Herb Categories

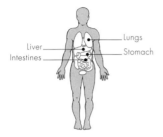

Liver
Intestines

Lungs
Stomach

Internal organs

Many diseases in TCM are attributed to energy weakness and imbalance in the body's internal organs.

One of the main divisions of herbal remedies is, as with ailments, into those used for treating "exterior" conditions and those for "interior" problems.

Exterior or superficial problems are the sort that we would describe in the West as minor or self-limiting. The group includes most common childhood disorders (such as measles or chicken pox), as well as colds, the flu, or minor aches and pains. Many of the herbs in this group are the sort that we would describe as antibacterial or diaphoretic —remedies that encourage sweating to help reduce body temperature in cases of fevers.

Interior conditions are usually more severe and are, in Chinese theory, associated with internal imbalance that can have a number of causes. The herbs used for interior problems are often very specific in action and remedies are aimed at restoring inner balance either by stimulating some sort of vital energy or a body organ.

The remedies chosen will be closely matched to the disease syndrome identified by the practitioner. This could be associated with a particular organ weakness—such as liver or kidney deficiency—or may be an imbalance associated with poor metabolism leading to too much "phlegm" or "dampness." Organ deficiency is treated with herbs that have an affinity for the specific part of the body since they act on the appropriate acupuncture meridian. For a surfeit of dampness the patient may be given warm, drying remedies to help restore balance.

The Categories

Typical groups of herbs included in the following section are:

Herbs to Balance Yin and Yang (see pages 60–79)

Herbs to Regulate and Tonify Qi or vital energy (see pages 80–95)

Herbs to Regulate and Tonify Xue or blood (see pages 96–119)

Herbs to Clear Heat (see pages 120–143)

Herbs to Warm the Interior (see pages 144–155)

"Draining Herbs," which encourage waste products to drain from the body—these would be labeled as laxatives in the West (see pages 156–159)

Herbs to Clear Painful Obstructions— remedies that we might label as antiarthritic in the West (see pages 160–171)

Herbs to Clear Phlegm and Dampness (see pages 172–199)

Herbs for Essence—a substance similar to energy believed in TCM to be responsible for creativity and reproduction (see pages 200–207)

Herbs to Calm the Spirit—loosely comparable to Western sedatives (see pages 208–213)

More Information

For more information see **blood (Xue)**, pages 96–97; **essence (Jing)**, pages 100–101; **Qi**, pages 200–201; **types of Qi**, pages 88–89; **spirit (Shen)**, pages 100–101.

THE FIVE ELEMENT MODEL

Early Chinese philosophers believed that all life was intricately bound together and tried to explain the natural events they saw in the changing seasons through a simple model. Winter rains caused new green plants to emerge in the spring. These in turn were scorched by the heat of high summer, leading to forest fires that created ashes, and returned to earth. From the earth came the metal ores used by the early copper- and bronze-smiths, while the cold metal surfaces caused water to condense, so completing the cycle.

Organs and body functions

The Chinese philosophers' observations were developed into the five element model, which is central to Traditional Chinese Medicine. The five element model links the basic substances of water, wood, fire, earth, and metal but each one has its own appropriate season, direction, color, body organs, emotion, and taste. Each element supports or restrains those other elements that are connected to it in the model and the same actions are also extended to the body's various organs.

Weakened water (related to the kidney) can fail to control fire (heart), which then attacks metal (associated with the lung). Their cycle explains why, in some cases of asthma, a Chinese practitioner will declare that the kidney is weak and prescribe suitable tonics rather than concentrating on respiratory remedies.

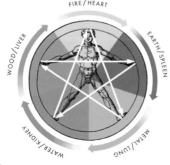

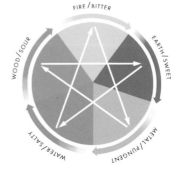

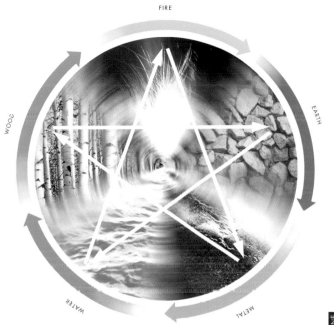

FIRE

EARTH

WOOD

WATER

METAL

Five element balance

Water controls Fire, while Fire will
control Metal. If Water is weak and
fails to control Fire, then Fire's action
on metal becomes excessive and Metal
is weakened as a result—this then
has an impact on the rest of the cycle.
Inevitably if one element fails to fulfill its
controlling/restraining duties then the
imbalance can become much more
severe and damaging.

Chinese Therapeutics

Traditional Chinese Medicine is generally aimed at restoring the inner balance and harmony of the body with remedies that will help to moderate any inherent "over-exuberance" or weakness among the five elements.

The various associations of the five key elements are a significant factor in any diagnosis. Colors, emotions, and tastes all link into the model, for example, an unnaturally red complexion on a person could suggest heart imbalance. Too much anger could hint at overactive liver energies (see the table, right).

Seasonal factors are also important. "Summer heat," for example, was blamed for the hot weather fevers that would have been common among ancient societies that lacked a modern understanding of hygiene and infection. Autumn in central China is usually associated with dryness, and lack of rain and water was linked to seasonal lung disorders with characteristic dry coughs.

The eight principles

Unlike Western physicians, TCM practitioners are unlikely to focus on bacteria or tissue damage to identify the likely pathology. Instead they will look at the basic pattern of the disharmony, which will help to pinpoint the cause of the illness. The first stage is to decide whether the problem is internal or external—caused by some inner imbalance or related to an external factor (see pages 36–37). Then the practitioner will try to identify the nature of any imbalance. That is, whether it is a problem associated with "cold" or "heat," if there is imbalance between the two great forces of Taoist thought —yin and yang (see pages 60–61)— or if it is a problem of excess or deficient inner energy levels.

This process is known as following the "eight guiding principles" or *Ba Gang* (the four sets of two opposites). Diagnosis is simply a matter of logically considering these possibilities and identifying what the underlying cause of the problem is.

The Eight Guiding Principles: Ba Gang

Deficiency	Excess
Cold	Heat
Yin	Yang
Interior	Exterior

Five Element Links

Element	Wood	Fire	Earth	Metal	Water
Direction	East	South	Center	West	North
Color	Green	Red	Yellow	White	Black
Season	Spring	Summer	Late summer	Autumn	Winter
Climate	Wind	Hot	Dampness	Dryness	Cold
Solid organ (Zang)	Liver	Heart	Spleen	Lung	Kidney
Hollow organ (Fu)	Gall-bladder	Small intestine	Stomach	Large intestine	Urinary bladder
Sense organs	Eyes (Sight)	Tongue (Speech)	Mouth (Taste)	Nose (Smell)	Ears (Hearing)
Emotion	Anger	Joy/fright	Worry	Sadness /grief	Fear
Taste	Sour	Bitter	Sweet	Pungent /acrid	Salty
Tissues	Tendons/ nails	Blood vessels/ complexion	Muscles/ lips	Skin/ body hair	Bone/ head hair
Body fluid	Tears	Sweat	Saliva	Mucus	Urine

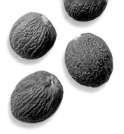

Rou Dou Kou

Rou Dou Kou (nutmeg) is a warming remedy often used for treating diarrhea and to warm the spleen and stomach.

RESTORING BALANCE
Just as illnesses can be defined in terms of their essential five-element associations, so too can plants. These remedies can then be used to combat the imbalance that has been causing the problem to restore harmony. A "hot" disorder, such as swollen inflamed joints or a fever, would be treated with cooling herbs, for example. An imbalance in the five organs, in contrast, could be countered by specific tonic herbs to help strengthen or control the organs involved.

Wu Wei Zi

Wu Wei Zi (schisandra) is used to replenish Qi, tonify the heart and kidney, and encourage secretion of body fluids.

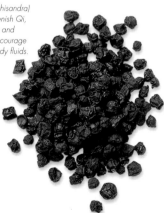

Western View

Western medicine might explain the effectiveness of Si Shen Wan (see box opposite) by arguing that nutmeg and Bu Gu Zhi (scurf pea) are also bitter astringents to relieve the symptoms of diarrhea and stimulate digestion. In addition, both Wu Zhu Yu (evodia) and Wu Wei Zi (schisandra) have antibacterial activity, which would help normalize gut flora and combat any infection contributing to the problem.

Si Shen Wan

Occasional diarrhea might indicate food poisoning. Habitual early morning diarrhea, however, is associated in TCM with cold and weakness in spleen and kidney energies. Associated symptoms are likely to include poor appetite, indigestion, and low back pain.

Si Shen Wan is often used to treat this sort of problem, and the key therapeutic ingredients of this are Bu Gu Zhi (scurf pea), Wu Zhu Yu (evodia), Rou Dou Kou (nutmeg), and Wu Wei Zi (schisandra). Additionally, Sheng Jiang (fresh ginger) and Da Zao (Chinese dates) help to harmonize the mixture and combat the slight toxicity of Wu Zhu Yu. Of the main ingredients, Bu Gu Zhi and Wu Wei Zi are used to strengthen kidney energy, while Rou Dou Kou and Wu Zhu Yu are warming remedies to clear cold from the spleen.

This whole combination therefore helps to combat the causes of cold and energy weakness rather than simply countering the symptoms as a Western allopathic remedy would do.

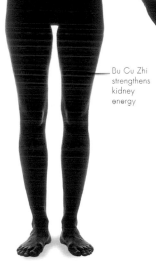

Rou Dou Kou and Wu Zhu Yu clear cold from spleen

Bu Gu Zhi strengthens kidney energy

Warmth and strength
Bu Gu Zhi (scurf pea) and Wu Wei Zi (schisandra) help to strengthen kidney energy; Rou Dou Kou (nutmeg) and Wu Zhu Yu (evodia) clear cold from the spleen.

Herbs for Exterior Conditions

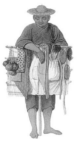

Damp
Elderly Chinese will still wear hats when outside in late summer to prevent an attack by damp, traditionally regarded as likely to assail the head.

Before the days of microscopes and microbiology, infections were blamed on some sudden external evil. In ancient China the dramatic seasonal changes of a continental climate were cast as the villains and the key "six evils" (Liu Yin) were defined as:
Wind (Feng), associated with spring.
Cold (Han), characteristic of winter.
Heat (Re) or summer heat (Shu), linked to high summer.

Dampness (Shi), most associated with the rainy season in late summer.
Dryness (Zao), typical of autumn.
Fire (Huo), associated with hot conditions, but while heat is a seasonal "evil", fire can occur at any time.

Characteristic patterns

These evils each had their characteristic symptoms, for example, fevers and chills from hot and cold or a shifting pattern of pain related to wind. An attack of dampness was characterized by runny phlegm or edema, while heat was the explanation for summer fevers. A cold spring was regarded by Chinese physicians as likely to herald cold-related disorders. These external evils can also attack in combination. Most common are wind-cold and wind-heat, perhaps with the addition of damp.

Herbs to combat evils

The major herbs for exterior conditions are classified into two groups: warm, pungent herbs for dispelling wind-cold and cool, pungent herbs for wind-heat.

Among the warm, pungent group are: Ma Huang (ephedra), Gui Zhi (cinnamon twigs), Zi Su Ye (perilla leaf), Fang Feng (ledebouriella), Qiang Huo (*Notopterygium incisium*), Gao Ben (Chinese lovage), Bai Zhi (dahurian angelica), Sheng Jiang (fresh ginger), Xin Yi Hua (*Magnolia liliiflora* flowers), and Cong Bai (scallions).

Herbs for clearing wind-heat are: Bo He (field mint), Niu Bang Zi (burdock), Sang Ye (mulberry leaves), Ju Hua (chrysanthemum), Ge Gen (kudzu root), Chai Hu (bupleurum), and Sheng Ma (bugbane, cohosh).

Children and TCM

In TCM, childhood ailments are regarded as simple exterior conditions. Only herbs suggested for exterior conditions should be used at home. Give one-quarter of the adult dose for children aged 3–4 increasing to one-half by age 9–10. For very young children seek professional guidance.

MA HUANG Ephedra

Ma Huang is the original source of the drug ephedrine that is used in asthmatic and phlegmy conditions. Shen Nong listed it as a remedy for malaria and headaches while Tao Hong Jing, in the sixth century AD, recommended it as "the first choice in treating cold damage." Today it is mainly used for external or superficial problems, especially wind-cold. The root (Ma Huang Gen) is an astringent used for abnormal sweating associated with internal deficiencies.

At A Glance

BOTANICAL NAME
Ephedra sinica

COMMON NAMES
Ephedra, Joint fir

FAMILY
Ephedraceae

PARTS USED
Twigs or stems

TASTE
Pungent, slightly bitter

CHARACTER
Warm

MERIDIANS
Lung, urinary bladder

ACTIONS
Antispasmodic, antibacterial, antiviral, induces sweating, stimulates urine flow, reduces fever

TRADITIONAL USES
- for excessive superficial syndromes due to wind-cold
- to encourage sweating
- to mobilize lung Qi
- to increase urination

TYPICAL CHINESE DOSE
7/100–¼ ounce (2–6 grams)

COMBINATIONS
Used with Gui Zhi (cinnamon twigs) for wind-cold problems. Often used with Xing Ren (apricot seeds) and Gan Cao (licorice root) for asthma and breathing difficulties associated with lung Qi stagnation; with Huang Qin (baical skullcap), Sang Bai Pi (mulberry root bark), and Shi Gao (gypsum) for heat obstructing the lungs; and also with Gan Jiang (dried ginger) for congested body fluids.

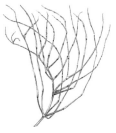

EPHEDRA

Cautions

Avoid in insomnia, deficiency syndromes (see pages 68–69), or raised blood pressure. Legally restricted in many Western countries due to the toxicity of ephedrine.

GUI ZHI Cinnamon

Both the twigs (Gui Zhi) and bark (Rou Gui) are used medicinally. The bark is considered to be the hotter of the two and affects central parts of the body, while Gui Zhi is seen as warming the exterior and peripheries—in the same way that twigs represent the outermost parts of the tree. Gui Zhi first appeared in a Tang Dynasty herbal in around 660AD and is considered to be less strong than Ma Huang (ephedra).

At A Glance

BOTANICAL NAME
Cinnamomum cassia

COMMON NAMES
Cinnamon, cassia

FAMILY
Lauraceae

PART USED
Twigs

TASTE
Pungent, sweet

CHARACTER
Warm

MERIDIANS
Heart, lung, urinary bladder

ACTIONS
Antibacterial, antifungal, antiviral, analgesic, relieves gas and indigestion, improves heart function, stimulates urine flow

TRADITIONAL USES
• to warm the channels and collaterals
• to disperse cold
• to improve circulation of yang Qi
• to strengthen heart yang

TYPICAL CHINESE DOSE
⅒–⅓ ounce (3–9 grams)

COMBINATIONS
Often used with Ma Huang (ephedra) for exterior cold, such as common colds and arthritic problems. Used with Fu Ling (tuckahoe), Gan Cao (licorice root), or Dan Shen (Chinese sage) for various heart-related problems, including angina pectoris, and with Wu Zhu Yu (evodia) for abdominal and period pains associated with cold.

CINNAMON

Cautions

Avoid in feverish conditions, excess heat or fire, and throughout pregnancy.

Diagnosing Exterior Conditions

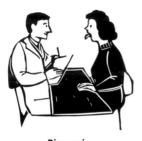

Diagnosis
The appearance—color, texture, and shape—of the tongue is an important diagnostic guide in Chinese medicine.

Early Chinese physicians had to depend on what they could see, smell, hear, and feel. The four stages of diagnosis are still used in TCM today:
• inspection of the patient's appearance, tongue, nose, skin color, and so on;
• ausculation and olfaction (hearing and smelling), which includes listening to the patient's voice and breathing rhythms and smelling any body odors;
• asking detailed questions about both symptoms and general well-being;

• palpation, which includes the complexities of Chinese pulse-taking, as well as feeling the body surface.

Spotting the superficial
Superficial or exterior syndromes, which largely affect the exterior of the body, include the majority of children's self-limiting ailments as well as problems such as the common cold. In the West these would be blamed on invading pathogens (viruses or bacteria) and are associated with the usual signs of infection such as raised temperature, fever, or chills. Depending on the mix of symptoms the Chinese practitioner will identify which of the external evils is to blame: cold conditions are obviously typified by feeling cold and having a pale complexion, while hot conditions include sweating and feeling hot. If wind is involved the symptoms will be shifting, like the wind. For example, rheumatic twinges and assorted aches are often associated with wind attack.

Lesser evils

As well as the six main "evils," exterior or superficial conditions can also be caused by other factors:

• improper diet, since food is the source of vital energy;

• fatigue that consumes vital energy (Qi), so weakening the body;

• inactivity and too much leisure time, which slows down energy and blood circulation and leads to stagnation and dysfunction of the spleen and stomach;

• sexual indulgence that damages reproductive energies and the kidneys;

• trauma and accidents;

• epidemics causing plagues (now a rarity thanks to better public hygiene and heath care);

• insect and animal bites.

Observation

"The skillful doctor knows by observation, the mediocre doctor by interrogation, the ordinary doctor by palpation."
Zhang Zhongjing c. 150–219AD

GAO BEN Chinese lovage

This plant is closely related to the lovage, which is used as a culinary seasoning in the West. Gao Ben is widely used for menstrual problems and after childbirth, although its main medicinal uses are to treat chills and for pain relief. The herb was listed by Shen Nong as being useful for headaches associated with wind as well as helping to "render the facial complexion attractive."

At A Glance

BOTANICAL NAME
Ligusticum sinense

COMMON NAME
Chinese lovage, straw weed

FAMILY
Umbelliferae/Apiaceae

PARTS USED
Root and rhizome

TASTE
Pungent

CHARACTER
Warm

MERIDIANS
Urinary bladder

ACTIONS
Antifungal, analgesic, antispasmodic

TRADITIONAL USES
• to clear wind-cold symptoms
• to clear various wind-damp symptoms

TYPICAL CHINESE DOSE
$^7/_{100}$–$^1/_3$ ounce (2–10 grams)

COMBINATIONS
Used with Chuan Xiong (Sichuan lovage) and other warming herbs for pain at the top of the head; with Wu Zhu Yu (evodia) and Xiao Hui Xiang (fennel) for abdominal pains associated with cold-damp, and with Cang Zhu (gray atractylodes) for back and joint pains.

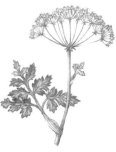

CHINESE LOVAGE

Cautions

Avoid where there is internal heat due to yin deficiency (see pages 68–69).

BAI ZHI

Dahurian angelica Bai Zhi is one of the several varieties of angelica that are used in Chinese medicine. It was listed by Shen Nong as a key remedy for vaginal discharges as well as being a specific for combating wind problems that are associated with head pains and watery eyes. He gave an alternative name of Fang Ziang, which means fragrance, for the plant, while Bai Zhi is usually literally translated as "white paper."

At A Glance

BOTANICAL NAME
Angelica anomala

COMMON NAME
Dahurian angelica

FAMILY
Umbelliferae/Apiaceae

PART USED
Root

TASTE
Pungent

CHARACTER
Warm

MERIDIANS
Lung, stomach

ACTIONS
Antibacterial, analgesic, induces sweating

TRADITIONAL USES
• to clear wind, especially in wind cold syndromes
• to remove pus and bring down swellings
• to relieve pain and headaches
• to dry dampness

TYPICAL CHINESE DOSE
1/10–1/3 ounce (3–9 grams)

COMBINATIONS
Used with Cang Er Zi (cocklebur) and Xin Yi Hua (Magnolia liliiflora flowers) for wind-cold associated with nasal mucus; with Chuan Xiong (Sichuan lovage) for pain and headaches, especially frontal pain; and with Bai Zhu (white atractylodes) and Zhe Bei Mu (fritillary) to combat boils and toxic swellings.

DAHURIAN ANGELICA

Cautions
Avoid if there is any evidence of stagnant heat syndromes linked with a yin deficiency (see pages 68–69).

51

Wind-cold Syndromes

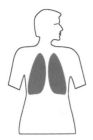

Lungs
The lungs are sometimes affected by exterior conditions moving to the interior.

Both wind-cold and wind-heat could be classified in the West as variants of common colds, minor respiratory infection, muscular aches and pains, and the flu, but in TCM they are each treated differently.

Wind-cold is typified by severe chilliness, slight feverishness, absence of sweating, headache, pains elsewhere in the body, a thin white coating to the tongue, and a pulse that feels as though it is floating. In addition, sufferers may complain of coughs or breathing problems.

In addition to common colds, wind-cold can also be blamed for swellings, boils, asthma, neck pains, and headaches.

Warm, acrid herbs are used to treat wind-cold. These are usually combined in decoctions, which need be no more than the familiar ginger and cinnamon tea. Simmer 1–2 slices of fresh ginger root in a cup of water for 10 minutes. Then add a pinch of powdered cinnamon, strain the mixture, and drink it three times daily. Gui Zhi (cinnamon twigs) is preferable to the variety normally used in Western cooking, although this is an adequate substitute.

Gui Zhi Tang

A more traditional Chinese remedy for wind-cold is Gui Zhi Tang:

Gui Zhi (cinnamon twigs) ¼ ounce (6 grams);

Bai Shao Yao (white peony) ¼ ounce (6 grams);

Sheng Jiang (fresh ginger) ⅒ ounce (3 grams);

Gan Cao (licorice root) ⅒ ounce (3 grams);

Da Zao (Chinese dates) ⅒ ounce (3 grams).

Xing Su San

This remedy for wind-cold is helpful if there is an associated coughing with thin sputum or thin, watery phlegm.

Xing Ren (apricot seeds), ¼ ounce (6 grams);

Zi Su Ye (perilla leaf), ¼ ounce (6 grams);

Zhi Ke (ripe bitter orange), ¼ ounce (6 grams);

Jie Geng (balloon flower) ¼ ounce (6 grams);

Chen Pi (tangerine peel) ¼ ounce (6 grams);

Ban Xia (pinellia) ¼ ounce (6 grams);

Fu Ling (tuckahoe) ⅓ ounce (9 grams);

Sheng Jiang ⅒ ounce (3 grams);

Gan Cao ⅒ ounce (3 grams);

Da Zao 3 pieces.

These herbs are traditionally combined as powders, although they could be made into a Tang sufficient for one day's doses. If diarrhea and abdominal fullness were also evident, then 1/10–1/4 ounce (3–6 grams) of Hou Po (bark of *Magnolia officinalis*) and Cang Zhu (gray atractylodes) could be added.

BO HE Field mint

This plant is traditionally used in the West to make mint tea and is added to milk to prevent it from curdling. In China Bo He is regarded as a prime remedy for superficial "wind-heat" problems, such as feverish colds, irritant skin rashes, or the early stages of the flu. It has been used medicinally for 1,500 years and was listed originally in the *Lei Gong Pao Zhi Lun* (*Grandfather Lei's Discussion of Herb Preparations*), which was written by Lei Xiao around 470AD.

At A Glance

BOTANICAL NAME
Mentha arvensis

COMMON NAME
Field mint

FAMILY
Labiatae/Lamiaceae

PARTS USED
Aerial parts

TASTE
Pungent

CHARACTER
Cool

MERIDIANS
Liver, lung

ACTIONS
Antibacterial, anti-inflammatory, antispasmodic, analgesic, induces sweating

TRADITIONAL USES
• disperses wind and heat evils
• clears the head and eyes and gives good spirit
• encourages the eruption of skin rashes as in measles
• disperses stagnant liver Qi and relieves depression

TYPICAL CHINESE DOSE
$^7/_{100}$–¼ ounce (2–6 grams)

COMBINATIONS
Used with Lian Qiao (forsythia), Jin Yin Hua (honeysuckle), and other herbs in the classic formula Yin Qiao San, which is a basic remedy for wind-heat syndromes. It is also mixed with Ju Hua (chrysanthemum), Niu Bang Zi (burdock), and other herbs to treat headaches and sore eyes associated with wind problems.

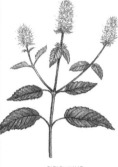

FIELD MINT

Cautions

Avoid in yin deficiency (see pages 68–69) and cases of excess liver Qi.

NIU BANG ZI Burdock

Burdock is familiar in the West as a cleansing remedy for skin and arthritic conditions. The leaves and roots are used in European herbal medicine but the Chinese only use the seeds. They were first listed in an eleventh-century Chinese herbal and are today mainly used for wind-heat syndromes such as common colds, as well as throat inflammations, tonsillitis, mumps, measles, abscesses, and carbuncles.

At A Glance

BOTANICAL NAME
Arctium lappa

COMMON NAME
Burdock

FAMILY
Compositae/Asteraceae

PART USED
Seeds

TASTE
Pungent, bitter

CHARACTER
Cold

MERIDIANS
Lung, stomach

ACTIONS
Antibacterial, antifungal, stimulates urine flow, lowers blood sugar levels, lowers blood pressure, purgative

TRADITIONAL USES
• to dispel wind and heat in the exterior
• to detoxify fire poisons
• to speed the formation and resolution of skin eruptions, in infections like measles
• to moisten the intestines

TYPICAL CHINESE DOSE
1/10–1/3 ounce (3–10 grams)

COMBINATIONS
Used with herbs such as Jin Yin Hua (honeysuckle), Lian Qiao (forsythia), and Jie Geng (balloon flower) for wind-heat problems; with Ge Gen (kudzu root), Bo He (field mint), and other herbs for treating measles and irritant skin problems associated with wind-heat conditions; and with Ju Hua (chrysanthemum) for boils and infected swellings.

BURDOCK

Cautions

Avoid if experiencing diarrhea.

Wind-heat Syndromes

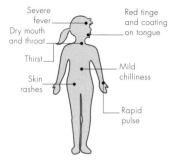

Severe fever
Dry mouth and throat
Thirst
Skin rashes
Red tinge and coating on tongue
Mild chilliness
Rapid pulse

Complex symptoms

Wind-heat syndromes can produce a mixture of symptoms that in Western terms would be usually associated with childhood infections like measles.

Wind-heat symptoms are complex and involve the likelihood of skin rashes as well as a fever. Many childhood infections such as German measles, chicken pox, and measles are in this wind-heat category. Typical symptoms include: mild chilliness, severe fever, a dry mouth and throat as well as thirst, a red tinge to the tip and edges of the tongue (which also has a thin yellow coating), and a pulse that is floating but more rapid than usual. There might also be skin rashes, as in measles. Wind-heat ailments can also manifest as more chronic conditions such as eczema or acne.

Yin Qiao Tang

For wind-heat problems a typical prescription would be Yin Qiao Tang, sometimes made into a powder (Yin Qiao San). This remedy contains:

Jin Yin Hua (honeysuckle) ⅓ ounce (9 grams);

Lian Qiao (forsythia) ⅓ ounce (9 grams);

Niu Bang Zi (burdock) ¼ ounce (6 grams);

Bo He (field mint) ¹⁄₁₀ ounce (3 grams)—added just before the decoction is ready;

Ban Lang Gen (woad root) ⅓ ounce (9 grams);

Xuan Shen (ningpo figwort) ¼ ounce (6 grams);

Jie Geng (balloon flower) ¼ ounce (6 grams);

Dan Zhu Ye (*Lophatherum gracile*), ¹⁄₁₀ ounce (3 grams);

Dan Dou Chi (fermented soybean seeds) ⅓ ounce (9 grams);

Gan Cao (licorice root) ¹⁄₁₀ ounce (3 grams).

Jing Jie (*Schizonepeta tenuifolia*), a wind-cold remedy, could also be added to warm the remedy. Herbs like Zhe Bei Mu (fritillary), ¼ ounce/6 grams, could be added if there was a severe cough, or Ge Gen (kudzu root) ¼ ounce/6 grams, and Huang Qin (baical skullcap), ¼ ounce/6 grams, might be included to combat high fevers and headaches.

Other sorts of common colds

As well as wind-cold or wind-heat, the symptoms of a cold or minor infection might also be blamed on seasonal "evils," such as a combination of summer heat and dampness. Internal factors can also play a part since weakened vital energy makes the sufferer more susceptible to attack from external factors.

More Information

For more information see: **Bo He,** page 54; **Gan Cao,** page 90; **Ge Gen,** page 59; **Huang Qin,** page 135; **Jie Geng,** page 191; **Jin Yin Hua,** page 142; **Lian Qiao,** page 143; **Niu Bang Zi,** page 55; **Xuan Shen,** page 131; **Zhe Bei Mu,** page 195.

JU HUA

Chrysanthemum Ju Hua are the flowerheads of chrysanthemums. They are used to make a popular cooling tea in China, which is now readily available from Chinese takeouts and supermarkets. The herb has been used for at least 2,000 years and was first listed by Shen Nong. He gave it the alternative name of Jie Hua (seasonal flower) and suggested that protracted use would "slow aging and prolong life."

At A Glance

BOTANICAL NAME
Dendranthema x grandiflorum

COMMON NAME
Chrysanthemum

FAMILY
Compositae/Asteraceae

PARTS USED
Flowers

TASTE
Pungent, sweet, bitter

CHARACTER
Cool

MERIDIANS
Lung, liver

ACTIONS
Antibacterial, antifungal, antiviral, anti-inflammatory, lowers blood pressure, relaxes blood vessels

TRADITIONAL USES
• to disperse wind and heat
• to clear liver heat and calm liver wind
• to neutralize toxins

TYPICAL CHINESE DOSE
⅓–⅗ ounce (9–18 grams)

COMBINATIONS
Used with Chuan Xiong (Sichuan lovage) for headaches due to external wind-heat; with Gou Qi Zi (wolfberry fruits) for headaches, dizziness, and vertigo due to ascending liver yang; and with Sang Ye (mulberry leaves), Bo He (field mint), Jie Geng (balloon flower), Lian Qiao (forsythia), and other herbs in Sang Ju Yin for alleviating the type of wind-heat that causes common colds and the flu.

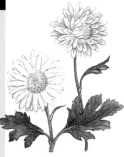

CHRYSANTHEMUM

Cautions

Avoid with diarrhea and in Qi deficiency (see pages 80–89).

GE GEN Kudzu vine

Although Ge Gen has been condemned as a pernicious weed in the US, recent research has highlighted its positive use in combating addiction, notably alcoholism. People taking extracts have been found to reduce their alcohol intake significantly. In Chinese folk medicine it is the flower rather than root that is preferred as a remedy for drunkenness, although Shen Nong recommends that the root will help to ease vomiting and clear various types of toxins.

At A Glance

BOTANICAL NAME
Pueraria lobata

COMMON NAME
Kudzu vine

FAMILY
Leguminosae/Papilionaceae

PART USED
Root

TASTE
Sweet, pungent

CHARACTER
Cool

MERIDIANS
Spleen, stomach

ACTIONS
Antispasmodic, circulatory stimulant, reduces fever, mild hypotensive (lowers blood pressure), and reduces blood sugar

TRADITIONAL USES
• to disperse wind-heat and wind-cold evils
• to raise the yang Qi
• to relieve skin eruptions, produce body fluids, and cool the body

TYPICAL CHINESE DOSE
³⁄₁₀₀–⅓ ounce (1–9 grams)

COMBINATIONS
Used with Bo He (field mint) for feverish chills and in the early stages of measles; with Shan Yao (Chinese yam) and Fu Ling (tuckahoe) for diarrhea associated with deficient spleen and stomach. It can also be used with Ma Huang (ephedra), Gui Zhi (cinnamon twigs), and Bai Shao Yao (white peony) for wind-cold problems.

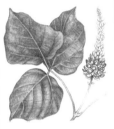

KUDZU VINE

Cautions

Avoid in stomach chills or if there is excessive sweating.

Yin and Yang

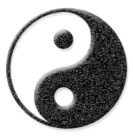

Balance
The traditional symbol for yin and yang reflects the presence of each in the other.

The Taoist concepts of yang and yin are now familiar in the West as alternating aspects of the creative force that is central to all things.

In traditional Chinese terms fire "defines yang" and anything that shares similar properties to this (warm, bright, light, moves upward, is active or exciting) is regarded as yang. In contrast, water represents yin—cold, dim, heavy, with a downward motion, passive, and inhibiting. Both aspects are, however, present at all times. While summer is more yang because it is a hot, bright season, it contains some yin. Damp and cold winter is closely yin but still contains a remnant of yang.

Yin and yang also apply to the human body so that substances (static things) are seen as more yin, while functions (activities) are more yang. Organs, blood, and body fluids tend to be yin, while the functions such as breathing and digestion are seen as more yang. Similarly the exterior is regarded as more yang, while the interior is more yin. The head (the upper part of the body, so is upward like fire) is yang and the feet (downward, like water) are yin.

Herbs for yin and yang

Weaknesses in yin or yang are usually related to particular imbalances in the organs. So, herbs that are used to tonify yin or yang are often organ-specific—helpful for deficient kidney yang, or deficient lung yin, for example. Many of these remedies are based on animal parts and would not appeal to

Westerners. Among the important yang tonics are Ge Jie (gecko), Hai Ma (seahorse), Hu Lu Ba (fenugreek), Hu Tao Ren (walnuts), Bu Gu Zhi (scurf pea), Yi Zhi Ren (*Alpinia oxyphylla*), Du Zhong (eucommia), Xu Duan (Japanese teasel), and Tu Si Zi (dodder seeds).

Herbs that tonify yin include Xi Yang Shen (American ginseng), Tian Men Dong (Chinese asparagus root), Mai Men Dong (lilyturf), Yu Zhu (Solomon's seal rhizome), Han Lian Cao (false daisy), Nu Zhen Zi (glossy privet fruits), Hei Zhi Ma (sesame seeds), and Gui Ban (tortoise shell). Some herbs, such as Dong Chong Xia Cao (caterpillar fungus) and Yin Yang Huo (barrenwort), can help both yin and yang.

Dawn until Dusk

"There is yang within yin and yin within yang. From dawn until noon, the yang of heaven is the yang within the yang. From noon until dusk, the yang of heaven is the yin within the yang. From dusk until midnight, the yin of heaven is the yin within the yin. From midnight until dawn, the yin of heaven is the yang within the yin."

Huang Di *Nei Jing*, c. 2500BC

DONG CHONG XIA CAO

Caterpillar fungus This fungus is a parasite that grows on a particular type of caterpillar, feeding on the animal and then fruiting in the spring. The traditional remedy used in China was actually a mixture of dead larva and fungus, although today Dong Chong Xia Cao is often cultivated on a grain base. In ancient China it was kept exclusively for use by the Emperor and his household and was cooked with roast duck to make therapeutic meals.

At A Glance

BOTANICAL NAME
Cordyceps sinensis

COMMON NAME
Caterpillar fungus

FAMILY NAME
Clavicipitaceae (fungus)
Lepidoptera (caterpillar)

PARTS USED
The whole fungus on the larva of *Hepialus armoricanus*

TASTE
Sweet

CHARACTER
Warm

MERIDIANS
Lung, kidney

ACTIONS
Anticancer, antiasthmatic, adrenal stimulant, antibacterial, sedative

TRADITIONAL USES
• to nourish the lungs and strengthen the kidneys and essence (Jing)
• to nourish lung yin and combat coughing

TYPICAL CHINESE DOSE
¼–⅓ ounce (6–9 grams)

COMBINATIONS
Usually cooked with duck, chicken, or pork as a tonic remedy for debility and weakened Wei Qi. It is also combined with Du Zhong (eucommia) and Yin Yang Huo (barrenwort) for impotence and lower back pains associated with deficient kidney yang, and with Xing Ren (apricot seeds) and other herbs for coughs and asthma.

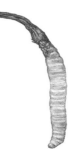

CATERPILLAR FUNGUS

Cautions

Avoid in exterior/superficial syndromes (see pages 44–45).

YIN YANG HUO

Barrenwort A literal translation of Yin Yang Huo is "horny goat weed." Modern research has confirmed it increases sperm production and stimulates the sensory nerves to increase sexual desire. Shen Nong recommended it for impotence and pain in the penis as well as noting that it strengthens Qi, essence (Jing), and determination or will (Zhi).

At A Glance

BOTANICAL NAME
Epimedium sagittatum

COMMON NAME
Barrenwort

FAMILY
Berberidaceae

PARTS USED
Aerial parts

TASTE
Pungent

CHARACTER
Warm

MERIDIANS
Liver, kidney

ACTIONS
Aphrodisiac, antibiotic, reduces blood pressure, stimulates urine flow (in low doses), lowers blood sugar, expectorant, antiasthmatic

TRADITIONAL USES
• to replenish vital function of the kidneys and fortify yang and essence
• to tonify yin and yang and control ascendant liver yang.
• to expel interior wind-cold-dampness

TYPICAL CHINESE DOSE
⅓–½ ounce (9–15 grams)

COMBINATIONS
Used with Wu Wei Zi (schisandra) and Gou Qi Zi (wolfberry fruits) for impotence and infertility associated with deficient kidney energies, and with Huang Bai (amur cork tree) and Zhi Mu (Anemarrhena asphodeloides) for menopausal problems.

BARRENWORT

Cautions

Avoid in yin deficiency (see pages 68–69) and fire syndromes. Do not use for more than 1–2 weeks continuously. Studies suggest high doses are toxic.

Balancing Yin and Yang

In a healthy body the relationship between yin and yang is constantly changing. If you exercise you become more yang, but rest indoors and you become more yin. These two energy forces also adapt to our changing needs in what the Chinese refer to as "mutual restraint," since each are controlling the other. In disease and illness, this mutual restraint collapses and imbalance in yin or yang follows. Herbs are used to help restore the balance, strengthening, or controlling these two elemental forces.

TCM defines four precise categories of yin–yang imbalance: overactive yin damaging yang; overactive yang damaging yin; excess yang resulting from a deficiency of yin; and excess yin resulting from a deficiency of yang.

Disease syndromes are defined in these terms and it is important to identify the nature of the imbalance in order to ensure accurate treatment: a disease characterized by inflammation and fever, for example, might be seen in terms of yang excess. But that yang excess could be due to overactive yang or simply because the yin is weak.

Diagram

Yin and yang need to be kept in healthy balance to maintain a person's well-being.

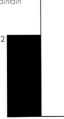
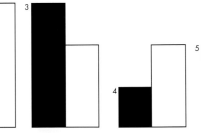

During the "observing" and "asking" phases of the examination (see pages 30–31), the physician is trying to identify what the state of the yin and yang is by looking at particular opposing characteristics. A yang deficient patient is likely to speak softly, sit still and quietly in their chair, or move slowly. If there is excess or strong yang then the person is likely to be more vigorous, moving rapidly and talking loudly. Complexion is also important. A pale, dull face suggests excess yin or deficient yang, while an over ruddy complexion can imply excess yang.

Diagnosis

Typical yin/yang characteristics that are used in diagnosis:

Yin	Yang
Hypoactive	Hyperactive
Inhibition	Excitation
Quiescence	Fidgeting
Pale or sallow complexion	Red or bright complexion
Soft voice	Loud voice

Key

The diagram opposite shows different yin-yang syndromes.

1 Yin and yang in balance

2 Excess yang: a hot excess syndrome

3 Excess yin: a cold, excess syndrome

4 Deficient yin: a hot, deficiency syndrome

5 Deficient yang: a cold, deficiency syndrome

6 Yin and yang deficiency

7 Yin and yang excess

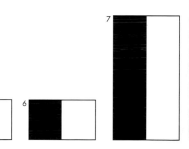

HU LU BA

Fenugreek This is a popular culinary herb that is regularly used in Middle Eastern and Asian cookery. Fenugreek is a very warming herb and is therefore an ideal remedy for treating all sorts of colds and chills that affect the abdomen, as well as acting as a yang tonic for the kidneys. In the Middle East the plant is known as *hilba* and it is used to counteract period pains and colic.

At A Glance

BOTANICAL NAME
Trigonella foenumgraecum

COMMON NAME
Fenugreek

FAMILY
Leguminosae/Papilionaceae

PART USED
Seeds

TASTE
Pungent, bitter

CHARACTER
Very warm

MERIDIANS
Kidney

ACTIONS
Antiparasitic, laxative, stimulates milk flow

TRADITIONAL USES
• to warm the kidneys and dispel cold
• to relieve pain

TYPICAL CHINESE DOSE
$\frac{1}{10}$–$\frac{1}{3}$ ounce (3–9 grams)

COMBINATIONS
Used with Xiao Hui Xiang (fennel) for hernia-like disorders as well as for period pains and with other kidney herbs, such as Bu Gu Zhi (scurf pea, see page 70), for pain and cold in the lower abdomen and back.

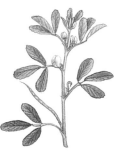

FENUGREEK

Cautions

Avoid if there are any fire symptoms, during pregnancy, or in cases of deficient yin (see pages 68–69).

HU TAO REN Walnut

In the West, walnuts are valued as a gentle nutrient and digestive remedy while walnut oil is a good source of essential fatty acids. The plant was first recorded by the Roman naturalist, Pliny (23–79AD) during a time when the nuts were regarded as the food of the gods. The plant has been used in China since the twelfth century and the nuts are regarded more as a yang tonic, and therefore especially helpful for the kidneys.

At A Glance

BOTANICAL NAME
Juglans regia

COMMON NAME
Walnut

FAMILY NAME
Juglandaceae

PART USED
Seeds (nut kernel)

TASTE
Sweet

CHARACTER
Warm

MERIDIANS
Lung, kidney, large intestine

ACTIONS
Astringent, anti-inflammatory, mild hypoglycemic (lowers blood sugar levels), laxative, nutrient (encourages weight gain), dissolves urinary stones

TRADITIONAL USES
• to reinforce kidney yang and strengthen the back
• to warm and strengthen lung Qi
• to moisten the intestines (acting as a laxative)

TYPICAL CHINESE DOSE
⅓–1 ounce (9–30 grams)

COMBINATIONS
Used with Du Zhong (eucommia) and Bu Gu Zhi (scurf pea) for lower back pain associated with kidney deficiency; with Ren Shen (Korean ginseng) and other herbs for asthmatic symptoms associated with deficient lungs and kidneys; and with Huo Ma Ren (cannabis seeds) and other herbs for constipation in the elderly.

WALNUT

Cautions

Avoid in heat, phlegm, or fire symptoms and deficient yin (see pages 68–69).

Deficiency Syndromes

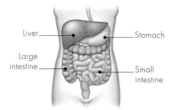

Digestive upsets

Deficiency syndromes can affect various organs. Spleen yang deficiency, for example, can be associated with digestive upsets.

Liver
Stomach
Large intestine
Small intestine

Deficiency syndromes can be caused by a weakness in yin leading to "hot, deficiency" problems, or to yang weakness, causing "cold, deficiency" characteristics.

Yang deficiency

Yang is associated with active energy and fire so a deficiency of yang energy leads to a lack of these sorts of characteristics. Tiredness and feeling cold are often signs of deficient yang.

It is important to ensure that the problem really is one of yang deficiency and not an apparent deficiency suggested by excess yin. Typical yang deficiency problems include an inclination toward recurrent infections with colds that never seem to clear, or a tendency to "catch everything around." Yang deficiency associated with specific organs can also be the cause of impotence (due to weak kidney yang), digestive upsets associated with weak spleen yang, or heart problems caused by deficient heart yang. When there is a yang deficiency, the therapy will focus on warm and tonifying remedies using herbs that are intrinsically hot.

Yin deficiency

Yin is associated with quiet and passivity so in yin deficiency these symptoms are diminished, which can sometimes create an appearance of yang activity or excess heat symptoms: restlessness, reddish complexion and tongue, and feeling warm or hot and feverish. Yin deficiency is often chronic and can be difficult to diagnose quickly or accurately.

Symptoms of yin deficiency include night sweats, sleeping problems, or an unnatural flush to the face. The pulse is likely to be fast and is described as "thready." Menopausal problems, for example, are often associated with liver or kidney yin deficiency.

While in the five element model the hollow (Fu) organs of the body are seen as yang, the major solid (Zang) organs—liver, heart, kidneys, lungs, and spleen—are defined as yin. Yin is also associated with fluid, so blood (Xue) and body fluids (Jin-Ye) are also predominately yin. Thirst and feelings of dryness can therefore suggest yin deficiency, similarly dry coughs can indicate weakness in lung yin and urinary problems suggest kidney yin weakness.

More Information

For more information see: **blood (Xue)**, pages 96–97; **body fluids (Jin-Ye)**, pages 100–101; **five element model,** pages 38–39; **Fu organs,** page 41; **heart,** pages 108–109; **kidney,** pages 204–205; **menopausal problems,** pages 204–205; **phlegm,** pages 172–173, 188–189; **spleen,** pages 176–177.

BU GU ZHI Scurf pea

Bu Gu Zhi is one of the main tonic herbs for yang and is therefore particularly effective for kidney energies. Traditionally it is used for "cock crow diarrhea," loose stools occurring in the early morning, which are seen as specific characteristics of spleen and kidney yang deficiency. The herb was first listed in the *Lei Gong Pao Zhi Lun* (*Grandfather Lei's Discussion of Herb Preparations*), which was written by Lei Xiao around 470AD.

At A Glance

BOTANICAL NAME
Psoralea corylifolia

COMMON NAME
Scurf pea

FAMILY
Leguminosae/Papilionaceae

PARTS USED
Fruit and seeds

TASTE
Pungent, bitter

CHARACTER
Very warm

MERIDIANS
Kidney, spleen

ACTIONS
Antibacterial, antitumor, astringent, uterine stimulant, relaxes coronary arteries, increases skin photosensitivity

TRADITIONAL USES
• to reinforce kidney yang
• to warm spleen yang

TYPICAL CHINESE DOSE
⅒–⅓ ounce (3–9 grams)

COMBINATIONS
For cock crow diarrhea it is often combined with Rou Dou Kou (nutmeg), Wu Wei Zi (schisandra), and Wu Zhu Yu (evodia). For back pain associated with kidney yang deficiency it can be used with Hu Tao Ren (walnuts).

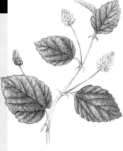

SCURF PEA

Cautions

Do not use if there is deficient yin or excess fire.

DU ZHONG Eucommia

Du Zhong was listed in Shen Nong's herbal as a remedy for pains in the lower back and knees and he suggests that long-term use may "slow aging." He gives its alternative name as Si Xian, which means "missing the immortal." Today it is considered an important yang tonic. First collected by Western plant hunters in the 1880s, the tree is the only surviving member of its genus. Extracts have been used to treat high blood pressure, and a decoction of the stir-fried herb is also particularly effective.

At A Glance

BOTANICAL NAME
Eucommia ulmoides

COMMON NAME
Eucommia

FAMILY
Eucommiaceae

PART USED
Bark

TASTE
Sweet

CHARACTER
Warm

MERIDIANS
Liver, kidney

ACTIONS
Stimulates urine flow, lowers blood pressure, reduces cholesterol levels, sedative, uterine relaxant

TRADITIONAL USES
• tonifies liver and kidney Qi
• smoothes the flow of Qi and blood to strengthen bones and muscles
• pacifies the fetus (to help prevent miscarriage)

TYPICAL CHINESE DOSE
⅓–½ ounce (9–15 grams)

COMBINATIONS
Used with Bu Gu Zhi (scurf pea) for lower back pains and breathing problems associated with deficient kidney yang, or with Gui Zhi (cinnamon twigs) and other warming herbs for problems associated with cold damp.

EUCOMMIA

Cautions

Avoid in deficient yin and active fire symptoms.

71

Excess (Shi) Syndromes

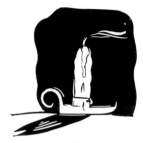

Dying Candle
The symptoms of excess yin are sometimes described as "the last flicker of a dying candle."

I n the same way as deficient yin or yang can lead to ongoing health problems, so an excess of either of these two vital forces causes problems too.

Excess yang

Since yang is closely associated with heat and fire, it is said to become "preponderant" when external heat or fire "evils" attack the body. Excess internal heat, believed to be caused by a range of factors including emotional imbalance, can further reinforce yang and so lead to disharmony. The system then goes into overdrive causing overreaction to stimuli, hyperactive metabolism, and an excitable personality. Typical symptoms include fever, thirst, and feelings of dryness, as the excess yang starts to damage inner fluids (associated with yin).

Predominant yang produces excess heat and if this is trapped within the body it can damage yin or, as TCM puts it, "excessive yang, hinders yin." This means that inner heat excess starts to manifest externally as false cold: yin on the outside of the body becomes disconnected with the overabundant yang inside, so body heat may be normal but the extremities are cold.

Excess yin

Excess yin conditions can be associated with attack by external damp and cold so that the body is unable to generate enough heat to balance the invasion. It can also result from a chronic yang deficiency rendering the vital energy incapable of combating external cold.

Preponderant yin leads to interior cold in the same way that excess yang leads to interior heat. This inner cold then inhibits the vital organs and impairs function. Yin excess is often seen in a pattern of abdominal pain, diarrhea, and "feeling cold." This interior cold causes blood vessels to constrict, impeding the normal flow and circulation, leading to pain.

Preponderant yin can then damage or "hinder" yang: the inner cold traps the yin inside the body so that there is an imbalance on the surface and an apparent yang excess or "false heat" is seen. External symptoms may include fever, thirst, and a red tongue.

Treating Excess Yin

First the excess level of yin must be reduced. Depending on the symptoms, this might require dry, warming herbs since yin is associated with fluid and moisture. Excess yin can, over time, also damage yang, so tonifying yang remedies would be given once yin is reduced. In excess yang, damp, cooling remedies would be used to reduce yang before yin could then be tonified and restored.

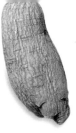

XI YANG SHEN American ginseng

This plant was "discovered" by Jesuit priests in Canada in the early eighteenth century and by 1765 it was included by Chinese herbalists in *The Omissions from the Grand Materia Medica* by Zhao Xue Min (*Ben Cao Gang Mu Shi Yi*). The plant rapidly became a valuable export. It was collected by frontiersmen like Daniel Boone and then shipped to China in huge quantities during the nineteenth century.

At A Glance

BOTANICAL NAME
Panax quinquefolius

COMMON NAME
American ginseng

FAMILY
Araliaceae

PART USED
Root

TASTE
Sweet, slightly bitter

CHARACTER
Cool

MERIDIANS
Heart, lung, kidney

ACTIONS
Improves heart function, hormonal action, sedative

TRADITIONAL USES
• to nourish Qi, fluids, and yin
• to nurture lung yin

TYPICAL CHINESE DOSE
⅒–¼ ounce (3–6 grams)

COMBINATIONS
American ginseng, like Korean ginseng, is often used on its own as a supportive tonic for yin and body fluids. It is also used for chronic coughs associated with lung deficiency and for fatigue and debility in chronic disorders. It is combined with Shi Gao (gypsum) for fevers associated with hot feverish conditions.

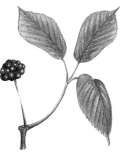

AMERICAN GINSENG

Cautions

Avoid during pregnancy and where there are symptoms of cold and damp in the stomach.

SHI HU Dendrobium orchid

Shi Hu, also known as *suk gok* from its Korean name, is a member of the orchid family. It has been used in Chinese medicine since the days of Shen Nong, who classed it among the "superior herbs" suggesting that it "prolongs life" and "fortifies yin." It also reputedly increases sexual vigor. Modern studies have shown that it lowers body temperature and is a mild analgesic.

At A Glance

BOTANICAL NAME
Dendrobium officinale

COMMON NAME
Dendrobium orchid

FAMILY
Orchidaceae

PART USED
Stems

TASTE
Sweet, slightly salty

CHARACTER
Slightly cold

MERIDIANS
Lung, stomach, kidney

ACTIONS
Mild analgesic, lowers blood pressure, digestive stimulant, reduces body temperature

TRADITIONAL USES
• nourishes yin and essence, clears heat
• nourishes stomach and lung yin and encourages fluid secretion

TYPICAL CHINESE DOSE
⅓–⁷⁄₁₀ ounce (9–20 grams)

COMBINATIONS
It is used with Sheng Di Huang (Chinese foxglove) and Xuan Shen (ningpo figwort) for fevers and muscular pains associated with excess heat; with Mai Men Dong (lilyturf) and other herbs for deficient stomach yin; and with Jin Yin Teng (honeysuckle stems) and other herbs for painful obstructions associated with wind damp and heat.

DENDROBIUM ORCHID

Cautions

Avoid in fevers that are not accompanied by dryness or thirst. Excessively high doses can cause breathing problems and convulsions.

Eating in Balance

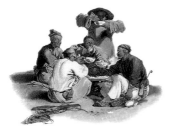

Yin–yang balance
The Chinese understand how the kinds of food we consume affect our inner yin–yang balance.

Just as herbs, parts of the body, and the seasons all have their particular yin and yang characteristics, so does food. Too many yin foods can cause yang deficiency or yin excess, while too many yang foods may mean the opposite imbalances arise.

Maintaining a healthy balance at each meal is an intrinsic skill that is important in Chinese cooking. Sour, bitter, and salty tastes are classified as yin while pungent and sweet herbs and foods are yang. Balancing these flavors is important to nourish both yin and yang. In the West we tend to eat far more pungent and sweet foods than we do sour or bitter ones.

In ill health a "cold" condition, such as a chill or watery diarrhea, should be treated with warming remedies and foods. A "hot" problem, such as an inflammation, should be treated with cooling dishes.

Matching foods to seasons

The ancient Taoists also preferred to eat cooling foods in winter so that the body would be in harmony with its icy surroundings. Hot spicy foods were preferred in the summer, as indeed they still are in many tropical countries.

For Westerners, coddled by central heating in winter and cooled with air conditioning when the temperature soars, these seasonal extremes have less significance: our climate tends to be fairly bland for much of the year. To match our neutral environment we should aim for an equally balanced diet ensuring that yin and yang, hot and cold, are in balance throughout the year.

Matching personal balance

Healthy people have their own bias in basic constitution; some are more yin while others are mainly yang. Some tend to feel the cold more. Others are hotter, and so may always feel thirsty.

A hot person should eat cold foods to help maintain an ideal yin–yang balance, while someone who is always cold should opt for warming dishes.

Hot and Cold Foods

Cold Foods bamboo shoots, banana, clams, crab, grapefruit, lettuce, seaweed, water chestnut, watercress, watermelon

Cool Foods apple, bean curd, button mushrooms, cucumber, lettuce, mango, mung beans, pear, spinach, strawberry, tomato

Neutral Foods apricot, beef, beets, Chinese leaves, carrot, celery, corn, egg, honey, polished white rice, potato, pumpkin, white sugar

Warm Foods brown sugar, cherry, chicken, chives, dates, ham, leek, mutton, peach, raspberry, shrimp, scallions, sunflower seed, walnuts, wine,

Hot Foods ginger, green and red bell peppers, pepper, soybean oil

HAN LIAN CAO False daisy

Han Lian Cao is one of the main herbs that is used in Traditional Chinese Medicine to nourish yin. It is an important liver and spleen remedy in Ayurvedic medicine and is also combined with other herbs in oils to combat hair loss and premature graying hair. In Chinese folk tradition this herb is used to treat skin problems, such as athlete's foot and dermatitis.

At A Glance

BOTANICAL NAME
Eclipta prostata

COMMON NAME
False daisy

FAMILY
Compositae

PARTS USED
Aerial parts

TASTE
Sweet, sour

CHARACTER
Cold

MERIDIANS
Liver, kidney

ACTIONS
Antibacterial, stops or reduces bleeding

TYPICAL CHINESE DOSE
½–1 ounce (15–30 grams)

TRADITIONAL USES
• to nourish liver and kidney yin
• to clear heat from the blood and stop bleeding

COMBINATIONS
Used with Nu Zhen Zi (glossy privet fruits) for severe deficiency syndromes characterized by blurred vision, tinnitus, prematurely graying hair, and dizziness. As a styptic (stops external bleeding) it is combined with appropriate herbs to stop various types of bleeding—with Ai Ye (mugwort), for example, for uterine bleeding; with Sheng Di Huang (Chinese foxglove) for coughing blood in deficient lung syndromes; or for blood in the urine associated with excess heat.

FALSE DAISY

Cautions

Avoid in cold and deficiency syndromes of the spleen and kidney.

NU ZHEN ZI

Glossy privet Nu Zhen Zi is one of the more important herbs used for nourishing the liver and kidneys that has been used since Shen Nong's days. He describes it as nurturing "the essence and spirit…able to eliminate hundreds of diseases," adding that it "prevents senility." Nu Zhen means "female chastity," a connection based on its pale green/white evergreen leaves.

At A Glance

BOTANICAL NAME
Ligustrum lucidum

COMMON NAME
Glossy privet, wax-leaf privet

FAMILY
Oleaceae

PART USED
Berries

TASTE
Sweet, bitter

CHARACTER
Neutral

MERIDIANS
Liver, kidney

ACTIONS
Antibacterial, improves heart function, stimulates urine flow, immune stimulant

TRADITIONAL USES
• to replenish the vital essence of the liver and kidneys
• to nourish deficient liver and kidney yin
• to darken the hair and improve eyesight
• to strengthen the knees.

TYPICAL CHINESE DOSE
⅓–½ ounce (9 15 grams)

COMBINATIONS
Used with herbs like Bu Gu Zhi (scurf pea) or Yin Yang Huo (barrenwort) for lower back pains associated with kidney weakness, and with Dang Gui (Chinese angelica), Shu Di Huang (Chinese foxglove), or He Shou Wu (flowery knotweed) to treat menopausal syndromes.

GLOSSY PRIVET

Cautions

Avoid if there is diarrhea with deficiency of yang (see pages 68–69).

Herbs to Regulate and Tonify Qi

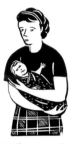

Family connection

Some aspects of Qi—our inner vitality and energy—are inherited from our parents.

Qi—sometimes written as ch'i—has become a familiar concept in the West over the past few years. Translated as "vital energy," it is understood to represent our inner vitality and energy—the substance that makes us tick. Its main characteristic is motion—the activity of life.

This is something of a Western over-simplification. In Chinese theory there are many different sorts of Qi. Some scholars suggest that up to 32 different varieties have been described in Chinese texts over the past 2,500 years as physicians have attempted to refine the definitions of these subtle energies.

Qi is basically a mixture of energies derived from the food we eat and the air we breathe. Part of our Qi is also with us from birth. These raw ingredients combine and are transformed in a variety of ways to make the different sorts of Qi that circulate within the body.

Qi is also seen as actual activity, such as the physiological function of body organs. Heart Qi, for example, is the action of the heart, not just an immaterial sort of energy state. Qi is believed to flow around the body, like blood, traveling in the acupuncture meridians and around the body's surface.

Herbs to regulate Qi

Herbs are used in TCM both to invigorate and energize deficient Qi and to move Qi around the body to avoid stagnation and to regulate the flow. Weak Qi is treated with tonic herbs, while sluggish or stagnant Qi needs remedies that help to move Qi through the channels.

Herbs to tonify Qi include Ren Shen (Korean ginseng), Dang Shen (asiabell root), Huang Qi (astragalus), Shan Yao (Chinese yam), Bai Zhu (white atractylodes), Da Zao (Chinese dates), and Gan Cao (licorice root).

Herbs to regulate sluggish Qi and combat stagnation include Chen Pi (tangerine peel), Zhi Shi (unripe bitter orange), Xiang Fu (nutgrass), Mu Xiang (kuth), Tan Xiang (sandalwood), Xie Bai (Chinese chives), Mei Gui Hua (Japanese rose), and Li Zhi He (litchi kernels).

More Information

For more information see: **Bai Zhu**, page 94; **Chen Pi**, page 82; **Da Zao**, page 95; **Dang Shen**, page 87; **Gan Cao**, page 90; **Huang Qi**, page 91; **Ren Shen**, page 86; **Xiang Fu**, page 83.

CHEN PI

Tangerine Chen Pi is the orange peel of ripe tangerines, while Qing Pi (green peel) is the skin of unripe fruits. The seeds, Ju He, are used for liver and kidney problems. Both these and Qing Pi are mainly used to smooth the flow of liver Qi and disperse stagnant liver energy, while Chen Pi moves spleen Qi. It eases abdominal discomfort, improves appetite, and is an effective expectorant.

At A Glance

BOTANICAL NAME
Citrus reticulata

COMMON NAME
Tangerine, Mandarin orange

FAMILY
Rutaceae

PART USED
Peel

TASTE
Pungent, bitter

CHARACTER
Warm

MERIDIANS
Lung, spleen, stomach

ACTIONS
Antiasthmatic, digestive stimulant, anti-inflammatory, relieves gas and indigestion, expectorant, circulatory stimulant; effective for acute mastitis

TRADITIONAL USES
• to strengthen and move stagnant spleen and stomach Qi
• to dry dampness and resolve phlegm
• to reverse the upward flow of Qi, and direct it downward
• to help prevent stagnation, especially when using tonifying herbs

TYPICAL CHINESE DOSE
1/10–1/3 ounce (3–9 grams)

COMBINATIONS
Used with Hou Po (bark of Magnolia officinalis) and Cang Zhu (gray atractylodes) for abdominal fullness associated with stagnant spleen and stomach Qi; with Qi tonics such as Dang Shen (asiabell root) and Huang Qi (astragalus) to balance the action of these remedies.

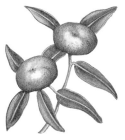

TANGERINE

Cautions

Avoid in heat syndromes associated with yin deficiency (see pages 68–69).

XIANG FU Nutgrass Xiang Fu

literally means "aromatic attachment" and this translation describes the highly scented plant perfectly. The herb, known as *motha* in Hindi, is also used in Ayurvedic medicine as a remedy for heatstroke and stomach problems. In TCM it is classified as being a Qi regulator and can be prepared with vinegar to enhance its pain-killing effects or with salt to help it moisten blood and fluids.

At A Glance

BOTANICAL NAME
Cyperus rotundus

COMMON NAME
Nutgrass

FAMILY
Cyperaceae

PART USED
Tuber

TASTE
Pungent, slightly bitter

CHARACTER
Neutral

MERIDIANS
Liver, stomach

ACTIONS
Analgesic, antibacterial, antispasmodic for the uterus

TRADITIONAL USES
• to promote the circulation of Qi and smooth Liver Qi
• to relieve menstrual and abdominal pains

TYPICAL CHINESE DOSE
1/10 - 1/3 ounce (3–10 grams)

COMBINATIONS
Xiang Fu is used with Chai Hu (bupleurum) for chest pain and distension associated with liver problems and with Cang Zhu (gray atractylodes) for indigestion, abdominal pain, and nausea. It is the main herb in Xiang Fu San, which also contains Chen Pi (tangerine peel) and Gan Cao, (licorice root) and is a warming remedy for both wind-cold and internal Qi stagnation.

NUTGRASS

Cautions

Avoid in cases of diarrhea with yang deficiency (see pages 68–69).

Wei Qi, or "Defense Energy"

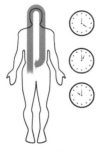

Wei Qi
Wei Qi circulates up the spine, over the head, and down the front of the body during the day.

travels through the skin and muscles where it controls the opening and closing of pores to regulate body temperature and moisten the skin.

Wei Qi movements

Wei Qi circulates during the day—traveling up the spine, across the head in the morning, down the front of the body during the afternoon to reach the lower spine at night, where it retreats back into the body.

This means that the time of any external injury is highly significant in Chinese medicine. A head injury in the morning, for example, is likely to damage the circulating Wei Qi and so will be more difficult to treat than a head injury later in the day.

Fu Zheng therapy

The traditional Chinese equivalent of stimulating the immune system is known as Fu Zheng therapy, which means "to strengthen" (Fu) "the constitution"

One of the main varieties of Qi is defense energy or Wei Qi, which is usually equated with our Western concept of the immune system. Wei Qi is seen as providing the main defense against attack from external "evils." If Wei Qi is strong, then the person is less likely to suffer from the sorts of colds and chills that the external evils might trigger. Wei Qi does not circulate in the blood but

(Zheng). Fu Zheng treatment can help to increase resistance to disease, prevent tissue damage, destroy abnormal cells, and regulate body functions. Allergies, lethargy, repeated infection, and slow wound-healing are all signs of lowered immunity.

Typical Fu Zheng herbs include Huang Qi (astragalus), Dang Shen (asiabell root), and Ren Shen (Korean ginseng) as well as many foods that are regarded as familiar foods in the West, such as shiitake mushrooms and seaweeds. Nowadays, these herbs are of value in combating the side effects of potentially damaging Western medical techniques such as chemotherapy and radiation, which can weaken the immune system significantly.

Seasonal Tonic

As a general seasonal tonic take Ren Shen (Korean ginseng) for a month in late autumn when the weather is changing from hot summer to cold winter. The body needs to adapt to the new environment during this particular time.

REN SHEN Korean ginseng

Ginseng is China's most important Qi tonic and it has been used for more than 5,000 years. During the seventeenth century a delegation from the King of Siam presented Louis XIV with a highly prized root of ginseng. The herb has been extensively researched and is now known to be rich in steroidal compounds that are similar to human sex hormones—hence its reputation as an aphrodisiac. It is also often used on its own as tonic to restore energy.

At A Glance

BOTANICAL NAME
Panax ginseng

COMMON NAMES
Korean ginseng, red ginseng

FAMILY
Araliaceae

PART USED
Root

TASTE
Sweet, slightly bitter

CHARACTER
Warm

MERIDIANS
Spleen, lung, heart

ACTIONS
Tonic, stimulant, reduces blood sugar and cholesterol levels, immunostimulant

TRADITIONAL USES
• to replenish Qi
• to tonify spleen and lung
• to generate body fluids
• to benefit heart Qi and calm Shen

TYPICAL CHINESE DOSE
1/10–1/3 ounce (3–9 grams)

COMBINATIONS
Used with Bai Zhu (white atractylodes), Fu Ling (tuckahoe), and Gan Cao (licorice root) in Si Jun Zi Tang for deficient spleen and stomach Qi linked to poor appetite, diarrhea, and vomiting. It is combined with Wu Wei Zi (schisandra), Sheng Di Huang (Chinese foxglove), or Mai Men Dong (lilyturf) for breathing problems linked to deficient lung or kidney Qi.

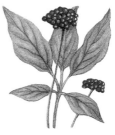

KOREAN GINSENG

Cautions

Avoid in heat and deficient yin conditions (see pages 68–69).

DANG SHEN Asiabell root

Dang Shen is often used as a less expensive alternative to Ren Shen (Korean ginseng). The herb is considered to be gentler and more yin than Ren Shen and is traditionally taken by nursing mothers. While Ren Shen (Korean ginseng) translates as "man root," Dang Shen means "relative root." It is a late addition to the Chinese materia medica, as it wasn't listed until 1751, when it was placed in the *Ben Cao Cong Xin* by Wu Yiluo.

At A Glance

BOTANICAL NAME
Codonopsis pilosula

COMMON NAMES
Asiabell root, Tang-shen

FAMILY
Campanulaceae

PART USED
Root

TASTE
Sweet

CHARACTER
Neutral

MERIDIANS
Spleen, lung

ACTIONS
Blood tonic (increases red blood cells), lowers blood pressure, immunostimulant, nervous stimulant, raises blood sugar levels

TRADITIONAL USES
• to invigorate spleen, stomach, and middle Jiao
• to replenish spleen and lung Qi
• to nourish body fluids (Jin-Ye)

TYPICAL CHINESE DOSE
⅓–½ ounce (9–15 grams)

COMBINATIONS
Often used as a substitute for Ren Shen (Korean ginseng). It is used with Huang Qi (astragalus) for deficient lung and spleen Qi associated with breathing problems and poor appetite; with Dang Gui (Chinese angelica), Shu Di Huang (Chinese foxglove), Bai Shao Yao (white peony), and other herbs for weakness associated with deficient Qi and blood. It is also cooked in soups and stews for deficient Wei Qi.

ASIABELL ROOT

Cautions

Avoid in attack by external "evils."

Different Sorts of Qi

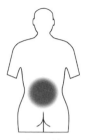

Yuan Qi

Yuan Qi is stored in the lower back, which is known as the gate of life in China.

There are many other types of Qi in the body. Some represent the inner energy with which we are born, but others are directly drawn from food and the air and can be adversely affected by poor diet and environment.

Primordial or Yuan Qi is with us from birth and reflects our parental inheritance. This sort of Qi provides the basic energy for the Zang-Fu organs and can be transformed into any of the other main types of Qi as required. It is stored in the lower back, which is an area called the "gate of life" in China.

Grain Qi (Gu Qi) is produced by the spleen from the food we eat. This then combines with "nature Qi" (Kong Qi), derived from the air we breathe, to form chest or Zong Qi, which is stored in the chest. Chest Qi fuels the circulation of blood and regulates heartbeat.

Primordial, grain, and nature Qi also combine to create normal or upright Qi (Zheng Qi). This spreads throughout the body and is the Qi referred to when the "Qi" of particular Zang-Fu organs is talked about. Zheng Qi warms and invigorates the body, it keeps blood and fluid in their appropriate channels, and can be subdivided into many other categories and functions.

Qi (Ying Qi) flows through the blood vessels, moving blood and supplying nutrients throughout the body. In cases of "blood deficiency," a Chinese physician will try to strengthen this Ying Qi.

Qi imbalance

There are four main disharmonies that can affect Qi: deficient Qi (Qi Xu), where energies are weak and insufficient; collapsed Qi (Qi Xian), when the energies are insufficient to hold the organs in place; stagnant Qi (Qi Zhi) where the energy does not flow smoothly through the body; and rebellious Qi (Qi Ni) when the Qi is moving in the wrong direction.

Daily Qi Flow

Each day our Qi travels through the network of channels in a well-defined rhythm. Any health problems with associated organs are therefore most likely to manifest at a particular time.

Time	Meridians
3–5 am	Lung
5–7 am	Large intestine
7–9 am	Stomach
9–11 am	Spleen
11 am–1 pm	Heart
1–3 pm	Small intestine
3–5 pm	Urinary bladder
5–7 pm	Kidney
7–9 pm	Pericardium
9–11 pm	San Jiao
11 pm–1 am	Gallbladder
1–3 am	Liver

GAN CAO Licorice

Shen Nong describes Gan Cao as one of china's most important tonic herbs. He say it is "sweet and balanced to treat the five Zang organs, six Fu organs, cold and heat, and evil Qi," adding that taking plenty of Gan Cao could prolong life. This herb is a valuable Qi tonic and, like Da Zao (Chinese dates), is often added to a prescription to help harmonize the action of other herbs.

At A Glance

BOTANICAL NAME
Glycyrrhiza uralensis

COMMON NAME
Licorice

FAMILY
Leguminosae/Papilionaceae

PART USED
Root

TASTE
Sweet

CHARACTER
Neutral

MERIDIANS
Heart, lung, spleen, stomach

ACTIONS
Antibacterial, anti-inflammatory, antispasmodic, antiallergenic, relieves coughs, lowers blood pressure, steroidal action, stimulates bile flow

TRADITIONAL USES
• invigorates Qi function
• clears heat and detoxifies fire poisons
• moistens the lung
• soothes spasms and relieves pain
• moderates the function of other herbs

TYPICAL CHINESE DOSE
7/100–1/3 ounce (2–9 grams)

COMBINATIONS
Used with Dang Shen (asiabell root) if the problem is to do with spleen Qi; with Xing Ren (apricot seeds) and Chuan Bei Mu (tendrilled fritillary) for dry coughs associated with heat; with Bai Shao Yao (white peony) for abdominal discomfort associated with liver weakness; and with Jie Geng (balloon flower) for throat problems.

LICORICE

Cautions

Avoid in excess damp conditions and hypertension.

HUANG QI **Astragalus** A Qi tonic
traditionally used for younger people. It is included in
Shen Nong's list of "superior" herbs as a remedy for
"pain, pus, and piles" as well as "hundreds of diseases in
children." Traditionally it is made into a congee (rice
porridge) for the Wei Qi. Recent research has confirmed its importance as
an immune tonic and it is also used for deficient spleen syndromes.

At A Glance

BOTANICAL NAME
Astragalus membranaceus

COMMON NAME
Astragalus, milk vetch

FAMILY
Leguminosae/Papilionaceae

PART USED
Root

TASTE
Sweet

CHARACTER
Slightly warm

MERIDIANS
Spleen, lung

ACTIONS
Antispasmodic, stimulates
urine flow, stimulates bile
flow, nervous stimulant,
antibacterial, lowers blood
sugar levels, lowers blood
pressure, immune stimulant

TRADITIONAL USES
• tonifies Qi and blood
• stabilizes Wei Qi and
stops sweating
• clears pus and
accelerates wound-healing
• regulates water
metabolism; clears odema

TYPICAL CHINESE DOSE
⅓–½ ounce (9–15 grams)

COMBINATIONS
With Ren Shen (Korean
ginseng) for debility, poor
appetite, and fatigue
associated with deficient Qi;
with Bai Zhu (white
atractylodes) for weakness
linked to deficient spleen Qi;
with Dang Gui (Chinese
angelica) for deficient blood
syndromes; and with Gui Zhi
(cinnamon twigs) for painful
obstructions and to strengthen
Wei Qi and nutritive Qi.

ASTRAGALUS

Cautions

In excess (Shi) syndromes
or if there is deficient yin
(see pages 68–69).

Qi-enhancing Techniques

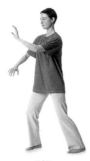

QiGong
QiGong is believed to "eliminate disease and prolong life" and uses exercises that strengthen and focus the Qi.

Traditional Chinese therapies include various exercise and massage techniques that are designed to strengthen inner energies.

QiGong dates back to the days of the Yellow Emperor and the Taoists. The name is derived from Qi—translated as "breath" or "vital energy"—and Gong (or Gongfu), which can mean the time spent acquiring a skill, the quality of the practice, and the actual attainment of the art. QiGong is translated both as "breathing exercise" or "energy skill."

This can be a useful form of self-help exercise for improving health and vitality, but it is also an important therapeutic technique. Traditional Chinese hospitals generally have a QiGong department where masters teach the technique to patients to help them combat chronic diseases.

QiGong massage

QiGong masters can also harness their own Qi for use in strengthening massage treatments for the severely ill. Massage therapy is also used to restore yin–yang balance: gentle manipulation and stroking are used in deficiency syndromes to restore balance, while in excess syndromes heavy manipulation is used to inhibit and reduce the surfeit. Yang massage includes energetic pushing, pressing, pounding, and knocking techniques while the yin group focuses more on stroking, smoothing, lifting limbs, or kneading.

Yang treatments are used to clear edema and swellings, to reduce pain associated with stagnation, and for insomnia. Yin treatments are used for Qi and blood deficiency, for general debility and weakness, or numbness associated with cold and dampness.

QiGong exercise

Mastering QiGong takes time. Experienced practitioners will often spend many hours holding a simple standing pose, focusing and controlling Qi throughout the body.

QiGong exercises are generally divided into three main groups: quiescent QiGong, a type of meditation; dynamic QiGong, which focuses on breathing routines; and dynamic-quiescent QiGong, which is probably the form most known in the West. It includes various postures and movement, or "training the body," and can look very similar to t'ai chi exercises.

Practice

As a simple self-help treatment for improving health and well-being QiGong takes practice. As the Chinese say, "the most important thing in doing QiGong exercise is perseverance."

BAI ZHU

White atractylodes Bai Zhu is one of the main Qi tonics that is used especially for spleen or stomach Qi deficiency syndromes. The herb has been used extensively in China since the Tang Dynasty (c. 650AD). It is used with Ren Shen (Korean ginseng), Fu Ling (tuckahoe), and Gan Cao (licorice root) in the famous "four noble ingredients decoction" (*Si Jun Zi Tang*). More recently, it has been promoted as a remedy to control appetite for use in weight-control regimes.

At A Glance

BOTANICAL NAME
Atractylodes macrocephala

COMMON NAME
White atractylodes

FAMILY
Compositae/Asteraceae

PART USED
Rhizome

TASTE
Sweet, bitter

CHARACTER
Warm

MERIDIANS
Spleen, stomach

ACTIONS
Antibacterial, anticoagulant, digestive stimulant, stimulates urine flow, lowers blood sugar levels

TRADITIONAL USES
- to tonify the spleen and Qi
- to clear dampness
- to control excess sweating and strengthen resistance

TYPICAL CHINESE DOSE
1/10–2/5 ounce (3–12 grams)

COMBINATIONS
Bai Zhu is mainly used for problems associated with spleen or stomach deficiency. It is used with Fu Ling (tuckahoe) and Chen Pi (tangerine peel) for deficient spleen problems; with Dang Gui (Chinese angelica), Bai Shao Yao (white peony), Huang Qin (baical skullcap), and Chuan Xiong (Sichuan lovage) as a blood tonic for menstrual problems; and with Gan Jiang (dried ginger) for cold conditions affecting the San Jiao (see pages 180–181).

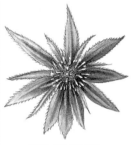

WHITE ATRACTYLODES

Cautions

Avoid in yin deficiencies (see pages 68–69) characterized by extreme thirst.

DA ZAO/HONG ZAO

Chinese dates Da Zao means "big date" and the fruits are one of the important "harmonizers" of Chinese medicine, often added to prescriptions to help modify conflicts in the action of the different ingredients. Da Zao are black while Hong Zao are red dates. The latter have a similar action but are regarded as more effective for nourishing blood. The usual method of taking dates is to add 3 to 10 to the Tang.

At A Glance

BOTANICAL NAME
Ziziphus jujuba

COMMON NAMES
Chinese dates, jujube

FAMILY
Rhamnaceae

PART USED
Fruit

TASTE
Sweet

CHARACTER
Warm

MERIDIANS
Spleen, stomach

ACTIONS
Nutrient, protects against liver damage

TRADITIONAL USES
• to tonify spleen and stomach Qi
• to strengthen nourishing Qi (Ying Qi) and blood
• to calm the spirit (Shen)
• moderates the action of other herbs

TYPICAL CHINESE DOSE
⅓–1 ounce (10–30 grams)

COMBINATIONS
Added to prescriptions to harmonize the remedy; with Ren Shen (Korean ginseng) to harmonize Qi; with Sheng Jiang (fresh ginger) for Wei Qi and nutritive Qi disharmonies and to improve digestion and absorption; with Gan Cao (licorice root) and Fu Xiao Mai (wheat extract) as a sedative for hysterical behavior associated with imbalance in the Zang-Fu systems.

CHINESE DATES

Cautions

In cases of excess dampness, food stagnation, or phlegm.

Herbs to Regulate and Tonify Xue (Blood)

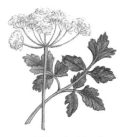

Nourishing the blood
A variety of herbs, including Dang Gui (Chinese angelica), can be used to invigorate blood circulation.

In keeping with TCM's pattern of fives, Qi is one of the five "fundamental substances" that are essential for life. The others are Xue (blood), Jing (essence), Shen (spirit), and Jin-Ye (body fluids); all are interrelated and can be nourished by the use of herbs.

Xue is a rather more tangible entity than Qi and is formed from a mixture of nutritive Qi (Ying Qi), food essence, and body fluids. On one level, Xue can be seen simply as blood, but it also has other attributes. In Chinese theory it is believed to be essential for mental activities: if Xue and Qi are strong, the person will be clear-thinking and vigorous.

Both Xue and body fluids (Jin-Ye) are yin. Body fluids are essential to maintain Xue so any loss can damage blood: sweating, for example, can damage Xue and lead to deficiency. In Chinese theory the liver is believed to "store blood," so any damage to the liver is likely to harm Xue with weak liver Qi leading to blood stagnation.

Blood disorders

In traditional Chinese pathology there are four major syndromes that can affect Xue: bleeding or hemorrhage; stagnant or congealed blood; heat attacking the blood; and deficient blood.

Herbs are used to "move" or combat these conditions. Styptic or coagulant herbs to stop bleeding include San Qi (notoginseng), Xian He Cao (Chinese agrimony), Di Yu (greater burnet), Huai Hua Mi (unripe pagoda tree buds), Ce Bai Ye (tree of life leaves), and Ai Ye (mugwort).

Invigorating herbs, such as Chuan Xiong (Sichuan lovage), Yan Hu Suo (bulbus corydalis), Jiang Huang (turmeric), Yi Mu Cao (Chinese motherwort), Yue Ju Hua (*Rosa chinensis*), Chi Shao Yao (red peony), and Dan Shen (Chinese sage), will move stagnant blood. Cooling herbs (like Chi Shao Yao) combat heat in the blood, and nourishing remedies, such as Dang Gui (Chinese angelica), help to build blood and relieve any deficiency.

In Western terms these four types of conditions equate roughly to:

• bleeding and hemorrhage;

• conditions involving clotting, such as thrombosis, as well circulatory problems and anything involving a build of blood or related tissue—as in the development of the womb lining before menstruation;

• irritant or inflamed conditions where the skin feels hot;

• anemia.

SAN QI

Notoginseng San Qi (also known as Tian Qi) is a close relative of the Korean ginseng and is used to clear any sort of blood clot or bleeding, such as swellings associated with traumatic wounds, soft tissue injuries, and bleeding. It is used in angina pectoris as well as in nosebleeds, abnormal uterine bleeding, and bleeding from gastric ulcers. The plant was first listed by Li Shi Zhen in his sixteenth-century herbal *Ben Cao Gang Mu*.

At A Glance

BOTANICAL NAME
Panax pseudoginseng

COMMON NAME
Notoginseng, pseudoginseng

FAMILY
Araliaceae

PART USED
Root

TASTE
Sweet, slightly bitter

CHARACTER
Warm

MERIDIANS
Liver, stomach

ACTIONS
Antibacterial, anti-inflammatory, improves heart function, circulation stimulant, stimulates urine flow, stops or reduces bleeding, lowers blood sugar levels, and relaxes blood vessels

TRADITIONAL USES
• to stop bleeding and clear blood stagnation
• to reduce swelling and relieve pain

TYPICAL CHINESE DOSE
7/100–¼ ounce (2–6 grams)

COMBINATIONS
Often used on its own but combines well with soothing Western remedies, such as slippery elm, for peptic ulceration. It is used with She Xiang (musk) in the formula Yun Nan Bai Yao, a potent emergency treatment for all sorts of internal and external bleeding. It is also used with Wu Bei Zi (nut galls) as a topical poultice for traumatic injuries.

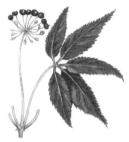

NOTOGINSENG

Cautions

Not to be used during pregnancy and only use with caution in deficient blood syndromes.

HUAI HUA Pagoda tree

The flowerbuds (Huai Hua), unripe buds (Huai Hua Mi), and fruits (Huai Jiao) of the oriental pagoda tree are all used in TCM to clear heat from the blood. The buds and flowers also help to lower blood pressure, while the fruits will clear liver fire. The unripe buds are less common in traditional medicine. They are a source of rutin, which is used in over-the-counter supplements to combat capillary fragility.

At A Glance

BOTANICAL NAME
Sophora japonica

COMMON NAME
Pagoda tree

FAMILY
Leguminosae/Papilionaceae

PARTS USED
Flowerbuds, fruits

TASTE
Bitter

CHARACTER
Slightly cold

MERIDIANS
Liver, large intestine

ACTION
Anti-inflammatory, lowers blood pressure, antibacterial, antispasmodic, stops or reduces bleeding, decreases capillary permeability

TRADITIONAL USES
• to clear heat from the blood and stop bleeding
• to cool the liver

TYPICAL CHINESE DOSE
⅓–½ ounce (9–15 grams)

COMBINATIONS
The buds are cooked with honey as a lung remedy. They are also used with Zhi Ke (ripe bitter orange) and other herbs for bleeding disorders in the lower part of the body, including hemorrhoids, and with She Xiang (musk) for vomiting blood. The fruits combine with Dang Gui (Chinese angelica), Huang Qin (baical skullcap), and other herbs in Huai Jiao Wan, which is used to combat blood in the stools and hemorrhoids.

PAGODA TREE

Cautions

Use cautiously in cases of cold deficient spleen or stomach syndromes or where uterine bleeding is linked to Qi deficiency (see pages 80–89).

Fundamental Fluids

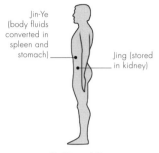

Jin-Ye (body fluids converted in spleen and stomach)

Jing (stored in kidney)

Jin-Ye and Jing

Jin-Ye (body fluids) and Jing (essence) are two of the five fundamental fluids essential for good health.

I n addition to Qi and Xue, the five fundamental fluids include body fluids (Jin-Ye), essence (Jing), and spirit (Shen). They are known as the "three treasures" and help maintain health and balance.

Jin-Ye

Like blood, Jin-Ye (body fluids) are yin in character. The name is derived from Jin ("clear fluid") indicating the clear aspect of fluid and Ye ("turbid fluid") suggesting the turbid or cloudy component. Jin-Ye

includes saliva, gastric juices, phlegm, tears, mucus, and sweat: all are seen as derived from our food and water and are converted in the spleen and stomach into the Jin and Ye.

Jin fluids are carried partly in the blood and also manifest as sweat. The thicker Ye fluids nourish the inner parts of the body such as joints, body orifices, brain, and bone marrow. Jin-Ye circulate through the body largely under the control of the spleen, lungs, and kidneys, so weaknesses in any of these organs may also be blamed for a resulting fluid deficiency or dysfunction.

Jing

Although Qi is more familiar to Westerners, the Chinese Jing or "essence" is even more important. It is the fundamental substance—the source of living organisms and the most important of this group of life materials.

Jing is stored in the kidney and comes in two types: congenital or innate essence inherited from our parents, and the acquired essence that is produced by the spleen from food, air, and water. The congenital essence controls both reproduction and creativity, while the "acquired" Jing reflects the quality of nutrition and lifestyle. The congenital essence is fixed when we are born and gradually runs down over our lifetimes. Its loss is associated with the physical signs of aging. Acquired essence—from a good diet and healthy lifestyle—can help compensate for weaknesses in our inherited Jing.

Shen

Shen is generally translated as "spirit," the inner strength behind both essence and energy. It is sometimes described as "awareness" and is also closely linked to lifestyle and creativity.

If Shen is damaged in any way then the person may be forgetful, slow-thinking, or suffer from insomnia.

More Information

Jing, page 200; Qi, pages 200–201; Shen, page 213; Xue, pages 96–97.

AI YE Mugwort

A familiar wayside plant in Europe, mugwort was once associated with magic and witchcraft, it is mainly used now as a digestive stimulant and sedative and is ideal for menopausal problems. In China, it is used for moxabustion treatments, where small tufts of herb are burned on acupuncture needles to warm the meridians. Studies suggest that, like its relative, wormwood (Qing Hao), it may also be effective for malaria.

At A Glance

BOTANICAL NAME
Artemisia vulgaris

COMMON NAME
Mugwort

FAMILY
Compositae/Asteraceae

PART USED
Leaves

TASTE
Pungent, bitter

CHARACTER
Warm

MERIDIANS
Lung, liver, spleen, kidney

ACTIONS
Antibacterial, antifungal, expectorant, uterine stimulant

TRADITIONAL USES
• to warm the meridians
• to stop bleeding
• to dispel cold and pain
• to resolve phlegm in coughs and asthma

TYPICAL CHINESE DOSE
⅒–⅓ ounce (3–9 grams)

COMBINATIONS
Used with E Jiao (gelatin from donkey hide), Shu Di Huang (Chinese foxglove), Dang Gui (Chinese angelica), Chuan Xiong (Sichuan lovage), Gan Cao (licorice root), and Bai Shao Yao (white peony) in Jiao Ai Tang—a classic formula for bleeding in pregnancy and threatened miscarriage. It is also used with Gan Jiang (dried ginger) or Rou Gui (cinnamon bark) for abdominal pain associated with cold.

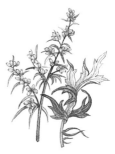

MUGWORT

Cautions

Do not use in cases of heat in the blood caused by yin deficiency (see pages 68–69). May cause epileptic convulsions in very high doses so is not to be taken by epileptics. Only use in pregnancy under professional guidance.

CHUAN XIONG Sichuan

lovage Chuan Xiong is related both to European lovage, largely used as a culinary herb, and to osha (*L. porteri*), which is a popular North American herb. It has been used in China since the fourteenth century as an invigorating blood remedy for menstrual and heart problems. It helps to ease constrained liver Qi associated with abdominal pain and is also an effective headache herb.

At A Glance

BOTANICAL NAME
Ligusticum wallichii

COMMON NAME
Sichuan or Szechuan lovage

FAMILY
Umbelliferae/Apiaceae

PART USED
Rhizome

TASTE
Pungent

CHARACTER
Warm

MERIDIANS
Liver, pericardium, gallbladder

ACTIONS
Antibacterial, lowers blood pressure, sedative, uterine stimulant

TRADITIONAL USES
• to invigorate the circulation of blood and Qi
• to relieve pain, headache, and skin eruptions caused by wind
• moves the Qi upward

TYPICAL CHINESE DOSE
⅒–⅓ ounce (3–9 grams)

COMBINATIONS
Used with Dang Gui (Chinese angelica), Bai Shao Yao (white peony), and Shu Di Huang (Chinese foxglove) in Si Wu Tang for menstrual irregularities and anemia. Also used with Ren Shen (Korean ginseng), Bai Zhu (white atractylodes), Dang Gui (Chinese angelica), and other herbs in Ba Zhen Tang for menstrual problems; with Chai Hu (bupleurum) or Cang Zhu (gray atractylodes) for indigestion and abdominal pain.

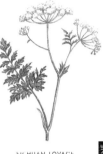

SICHUAN LOVAGE

Cautions

Not to be used for headaches caused by yin deficiency or over-exuberant liver yang. Avoid in pregnancy and menorrhagia.

Blood Stagnation

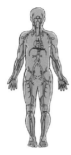

Circulation
In TCM the blood's circulation is believed to behave quite differently than our Western understanding.

The term "stagnant blood" is commonly used in TCM to explain a wide variety of heart and menstrual irregularities. The syndrome occurs when the flow of blood is blocked or the blood becomes static. Stagnant blood problems may be the result of external pathogens or be caused by inappropriate treatment of hemorrhage, by traumatic injury, by stagnation of Qi, or by retention of the lochia following childbirth. Stagnant blood is characterized by a fixed pain that is not eased by either hot compresses or ice packs. Other symptoms can include hemorrhage, while typical signs include purplish skin, dark purple lips, and dry scaly skin.

Thrombosis, local ischemia, certain heart disorders, menstrual problems, and hemorrhage might all be classified in TCM as aspects of congealed blood.

Menstrual problems

Many gynecological problems are associated with blood stagnation since the build up of endometrium (the womb lining) each month can be seen as a minor mass of stagnant blood.

Some sorts of period pain can be linked to blood stagnation, often with Qi deficiency or stagnation contributing to the problem as well. Symptoms include cramping pains a day or so before the start of a period, which is often irregular, and the menstrual discharge tends to be dark with many clots. Treatment would include using herbs like Dang Gui (Chinese angelica), Dan Shen (Chinese sage), Xiang Fu (nutgrass), and Chuan

Xiong (Sichan lovage), which help to invigorate blood and Qi circulation.

In TCM, chronic inflammation of the fallopian tube (salpingitis) is seen in terms of blood stagnation, linked to menstrual dysfunction. Again, treatment involves energizing blood circulation, easing pain, and stimulating liver energies. A typical prescription would be Shen Hua Tang, which combines Dang Gui (Chinese angelica) with Chuan Xiong (Sichuan lovage) and Tao Ren (peach seeds)—to invigorate blood circulation—with Gan Jiang (dried ginger) and Gan Cao (licorice root) to warm and harmonize the prescription. Xiang Fu (nutgrass) could be added to stimulate liver Qi, since liver energy is closely associated with menstruation, as well as Yan Hu Suo (bulbus corydalis) to ease pain.

More Information

Dan Shen, page 106; Dang Gui, page 115; Gan Cao, page 90; Gan Jiang, page 146; Xiang Fu, page 83; Yan Hu Suo, page 107.

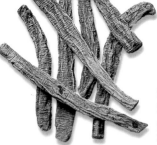

DAN SHEN

Chinese sage This is a heart and blood remedy that has been shown in clinical trials to help both heart disease and problems with cerebral circulation. It was included in Shen Nong's herbal as a remedy for "evil Qi in the heart and abdomen." He also gave it the alternative name of Que Chan Cao, meaning cicada-deterring weed. Dan Shen can also be useful for insomnia and palpitations, which may be related to deficient heart blood.

At A Glance

BOTANICAL NAME
Salvia miltiorrhiza

COMMON NAME
Chinese sage, Red sage

FAMILY
Labiatae/Lamiaceae

PARTS USED
Root and rhizome

TASTE
Bitter

CHARACTER
Slightly cold

MERIDIANS
Heart, liver, pericardium

ACTIONS
Anticoagulant, antibacterial, immunostimulant, circulatory stimulant, relaxes blood vessels, promotes tissue repair, sedative, lowers blood cholesterol, lowers blood sugar levels

TRADITIONAL USES
• to invigorate circulation and clear stagnation
• to clear heat
• to calm the spirit and soothe irritability

TYPICAL CHINESE DOSE
⅒–½ ounce (3–15 grams)

COMBINATIONS
Used with Dang Gui (Chinese angelica), Chuan Xiong (Sichuan lovage), and other herbs for period pains and irregular menstruation and with Mu Dan Pi (tree peony) and Sheng Di Huang (Chinese foxglove) for heat syndromes linked with nosebleeds or spitting blood.

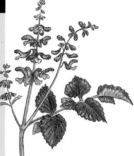

CHINESE SAGE

Cautions

Avoid using if there is no blood stagnation.

YAN HU SUO Bulbus

corydalis One of the most potent painkillers used in Chinese medicine. It is used for a wide range of painful conditions including period pains, lumbago, abdominal pains (including those caused by appendicitis and peptic ulceration), and traumatic injuries. The plant belongs to the poppy family—the source of morphine—and contains a similar strongly analgesic alkaloid called corydaline.

At A Glance

BOTANICAL NAME
Corydalis solida

COMMON NAME
Bulbus corydalis, fumewort

FAMILY
Papaveraceae

PART USED
Rhizome

TASTE
Pungent, bitter

CHARACTER
Warm

MERIDIANS
Liver, spleen

ACTIONS
Analgesic, sedative, antispasmodic, adrenal stimulant

TRADITIONAL USES
• to invigorate blood circulation to clear stasis
• to regulate the circulation of Qi
• to ease pain

TYPICAL CHINESE DOSE
⅒–⅓ ounce (3–9 grams)

COMBINATIONS
Used with Xiang Fu (nutgrass) and Chuan Xiong (Sichuan lovage) for period pains associated with stagnant Qi and blood; with Rou Gui (cinnamon bark) for period pains; or with Gui Zhi (cinnamon twigs) for pain in the extremities. It is also used for almost any sort of pain when combined with herbs that would help to treat the underlying condition.

BULBUS CORYDALIS

Cautions

Avoid in pregnancy.

The Heart

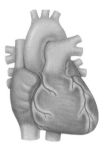

Heart
*According to Chinese medicine,
the heart controls mental activities as
well as the circulation of blood.*

The heart is classified as one of the
five solid or Zang organs of
Chinese medicine, along with the
kidneys, liver, spleen, and lungs. It is
described, much as in conventional
Western medicine, as controlling the
circulation or "governing blood and
blood vessels." Depending on the
heart's energy (Qi) the blood will be
vigorous and the person healthy and full
of life. As well as controlling blood
circulation, Chinese theory also credits
the heart with a number of attributes that

can seem quite alien to Westerners. For
example, it is said that it can be seen in
the complexion, be linked to the
tongue, and control mental activities.

The heart's close association with
blood vessels means that its health is
mirrored in the face. If heart Qi is
strong, the complexion is ruddy and
healthy. If the Qi is weak then the face
will be pale. The heart is also closely
associated with the tongue in the five
element model and so the Chinese
would argue that taste is a reflection
of heart Qi vitality.

Mental and spiritual attributes

The heart is said to be the ruling
member of the Zang-Fu organs and
controls all life processes. This is a
similar approach to other traditional
medical theories—including Ayurveda
and ancient Egyptian belief—in which
the heart is closely associated with the
soul and emotions.

In Chinese medicine, the heart rather
than the brain is seen as controlling
"mental activities," which is understood

to mean a wide range of thought processes, perception, mental health, and behavior. The brain is regarded simply as a system for receiving and storing information and so has no real involvement in thought processes.

Mental disorders are believed to be caused by some sort of damage to the heart, rather than the brain, and remedies that are traditionally said to "calm the spirit" are often ones which, in Western terms, we would use to regulate heart activity.

The heart is also associated with the emotion "joy." This is not entirely the pleasant emotion it seems. In traditional, conservative Chinese society, "joy" can also mean unruly or inappropriate behavior.

A Sick Heart

"Those who suffer from a sick heart are animated and quick-witted at noon, around midnight their spirits are heightened, and in the morning they are peaceful and quiet."

Huang Di *Nei Jing Su Wen* c. 2500BC

CHI SHAO YAO/BAI SHAO YAO

Red and white peony Confusingly, both red peony (Chi Shao Yao) and white peony (Bai Shao Yao) are variants of the same species. The names do not reflect the color of the flowers, but, with its darker roots, Chi Shao Yao, is traditionally collected from wild plants while Bai Shao Yao comes from cultivated specimens. Use of both dates back to around 500AD when they were listed in Tao Hong-jing's *Ben Cao Jing Ji Zhu*.

At A Glance

BOTANICAL NAME
Paeonia lactiflora

COMMON NAME
Red and white peony

FAMILY:
Paeoniaceae

PART USED
Root

TASTE
Sour, bitter

CHARACTER
Slightly cold

MERIDIANS
Liver, spleen

ACTIONS
Stimulates urine flow, anti-inflammatory, antispasmodic, sedative, lowers blood pressure, analgesic, anticoagulant, lowers blood cholesterol, lowers blood sugar levels, immunostimulant

TRADITIONAL USES
Bai Shao Yao: • to balance liver functions and energy
• to nourish blood
• to soothe liver Qi
Chi Shao Yao: • to invigorate blood and dispel stagnation
• to clear heat/cool the blood
• to clear liver fire

TYPICAL CHINESE DOSE
Chi Shao Yao: ¼–½ ounce (6–15 grams)
Bai Shao Yao: ⅓–⅗ ounce (9–18 grams)

COMBINATIONS
Bai Shao Yao is used with Dang Gui (Chinese angelica) and Shu Di Huang (Chinese foxglove) for menstrual problems associated with liver or blood deficiency.
Chi Shao Yao is used with Xiang Fu (nutgrass) and Chuan Xiong (Sichuan lovage) for period pains associated with blood stagnation.

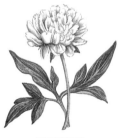

WHITE PEONY

Cautions

Avoid Bai Shao Yao in diarrhea and abdominal coldness and avoid Chi Shao Yao (red peony) if there is no evidence of blood stagnation.

HUAI NIU XI Two-toothed amaranthus

Huai Niu Xi translates as "ox knees from the Huai River." This may simply be a description of its knobbled stems but it also points to its use as a liver remedy. The liver is associated with tendons and, as there are many tendons in the knees, aching knees often suggests stagnating liver problems. Huai Niu Xi is a directional remedy, helping to focus attention on the lower part of the body.

At A Glance

BOTANICAL NAME
Achyranthes bidentata

COMMON NAME
Two-toothed amaranthus

FAMILY
Amaranthaceae

PART USED
Root

TASTE
Bitter, sour

CHARACTER
Neutral

MERIDIANS
liver, kidney

ACTIONS
Analgesic, stimulates urine flow, lowers blood pressure

TRADITIONAL USES
• invigorates blood circulation and clears stagnant blood
• strengthens sinews and bones, nourishing liver and kidney
• clears damp heat in the lower Jiao
• descends the flow of blood and Qi

TYPICAL CHINESE DOSE
¼–½ ounce (6–15 grams)

COMBINATIONS
Used with Du Zhong for pains in the back and lower limbs; with Dang Gui (Chinese angelica), Rou Gui (cinnamon bark), and Hong Hua (safflower) for menstrual problems associated with stagnant blood; with Dang Gui (Chinese angelica) and with Huang Qin (baical skullcap) for urinary problems such as cystitis.

TWO-TOOTHED
AMARANTHUS

Cautions

Avoid in pregnancy and menorrhagia.

Nourishing the Blood

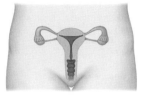

Menstrual cycle
In TCM the liver is believed to store blood, so is closely associated with menstruation and the menstrual cycle.

tonifying herbs to "nourish the blood." These herbs are often rich in nutrients, so they supply the essential minerals or vitamins that the body needs to build more blood. They are usually combined with yin remedies, since blood is a yin substance, so any deficiency is seen as yin weakness. Many remedies are used to tonify Qi and blood together since these deficiencies are often linked.

Deficient blood syndromes are characterized by pallor, dizziness, vertigo, poor eyesight, fatigue, palpitations, menstrual irregularities, deafness or tinnitus, and dry skin. A Western practitioner might blame some of these symptoms on anemia—an iron-deficiency common in women of child-bearing age—although they can also suggest heart weakness or possibly chronic liver disease.

In Chinese theory deficient blood symptoms almost always suggest problems with the liver, which stores the blood, or the heart, which directs and circulates the blood. Treatment uses

Period pain

While many menstrual problems are associated with blood stagnation, deficiency of Qi and blood is another common cause. Differential diagnosis is important; it would be inappropriate to nourish the blood if a remedy to encourage its circulation is needed.

Period pains associated with deficiency are characterized by a delayed start to menstruation, a dull ache rather than cramping pains, and a light-colored discharge without clots. The sufferer is likely to feel weak, tired, and may also suffer from palpitations and dizziness.

One of the classic remedies for this problem is the "decoction of eight precious ingredients" (Ba Zhen Tang), often marketed in tablet form as "Women's Precious Pills." This can contain Ren Shen (Korean ginseng), but Dang Shen (asiabell root) is often preferred since it is more yin in character, and more appropriate for blood deficiency. Other herbs used are: Bai Zhu (white atractylodes), Shu Di Huang (Chinese foxglove), Dang Gui (Chinese angelica), Bai Shao Yao (white peony), Chuan Xiong (Sichuan lovage), and Gan Cao (licorice root).

For blood and Qi deficiency, Huang Qi (astragalus) is often added with Rou Gui (cinnamon bark) or Sheng Jiang (fresh ginger) if a warming ingredient is appropriate. For irregular menstruation and back pain, Yu Mu Cao (Chinese motherwort) or a little Du Zhong (eucommia) are optional.

More Information

For more information see: **Bai Shao Yao**, page 110; **Chuan Xiong**, page 103; **Dang Shen**, page 87; **Dang Gui**, page 115; **Du Zhong**, page 71; **Ren Shen**, page 86.

HE SHOU WU Flowery knotweed

He Shou Wu (also known in the West as Fo Ti from its Cantonese name) is an important blood tonic that also helps to replenish kidney and liver energy. The Chinese name translates as "black-haired Mr. He"—a reference, perhaps, to its traditional use in restoring color to prematurely graying hair. It has been used as a remedy in China since the eighth century and first appeared in the *Ri Hua Zi Ben Cao* written in 713AD.

At A Glance

BOTANICAL NAME
Polygonum multiflorum

COMMON NAME
Flowery knotweed, fleeceflower

FAMILY
Polygonaceae

PART USED
Root

TASTE
Sweet, bitter, astringent

CHARACTER
Slightly warm

MERIDIANS
Liver, kidney

ACTIONS
Antibacterial, improves heart function, hormonal action, laxative, raises blood sugar levels, liver stimulant, reduces blood cholesterol

TRADITIONAL USES
• to replenish liver and kidney Jing and nourish blood
• to detoxify fire poisons
• to clear exterior wind
• to lubricate the intestines (as a laxative)

TYPICAL CHINESE DOSE
⅓–⅘ ounce (9–25 grams)

COMBINATIONS
Used with such herbs as Ren Shen (Korean ginseng) and Dang Gui (Chinese angelica) for chronic debility; with Gou Qi Zi (wolfberry fruits) and Bu Gu Zhi (scurf pea) for symptoms of premature aging linked to weak liver and kidney energies; and with Nu Zhen Zi (glossy privet fruits) and Huai Niu Xi (two-toothed amaranthus) for deficient liver blood.

FLOWERY KNOTWEED

Cautions

Avoid in diarrhea associated with phlegm or deficient spleen.

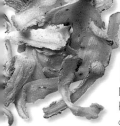

DANG GUI Chinese angelica

Dang Gui is one of the most popular Chinese tonic herbs in the West and appears in many over-the-counter products for gynecological problems. Shen Nong recommended it for malaria, coughs, adverse Qi flow, and "infertility in females." Different parts of the root have different qualities—the bottom tip of the root is said to move blood most strongly, while the uppermost part or "head" is a stronger tonic remedy.

At A Glance

BOTANICAL NAME
Angelica polymorpha var. sinensis

COMMON NAME
Chinese angelica

FAMILY
Umbelliferae/Apiaceae

PART USED
Root

TASTE
Sweet, pungent

CHARACTER
Warm

MERIDIANS
Liver, heart, spleen

ACTIONS
Antibacterial, analgesic, anti-inflammatory, circulatory stimulant, reduces blood cholesterol levels, liver tonic, sedative, uterine stimulant, rich in folic acid and vitamin B_{12}

TRADITIONAL USES
• to nourish blood and invigorate blood circulation
• to moisten the intestines and move stools (laxative)

TYPICAL CHINESE DOSE
$\frac{1}{10}$–$\frac{2}{5}$ ounce (3–12 grams)

COMBINATIONS
Used with Huang Qi (astragalus) and Sheng Jiang (fresh ginger) in lamb stews made to relieve postpartum pains; with Huo Ma Ren (cannabis seeds) as a laxative for the elderly; and with Bai Shao Yao (white peony), Chuan Xiong (Sichuan lovage), and Shu Di Huang (Chinese foxglove) for menstrual problems associated with deficient or stagnant blood.

CHINESE ANGELICA

Cautions

Avoid in pregnancy, diarrhea, or abdominal fullness.

115

The Liver

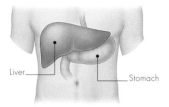

Liver functions

In TCM the liver has many functions, such as controlling tendons, which is very different from the Western anatomical view.

Liver

Stomach

I n Chinese theory, the key functions of the liver are to store blood and regulate the flow of Qi. While the heart governs the flow of blood, the liver stores it, regulating its release into the body as needed. This helps to explain why the Chinese associate the liver with the female menstrual cycle and will often treat gynecological problems with liver tonics.

The liver also regulates the way that Qi circulates through our bodies. The ideal is for a smooth and constant flow of Qi with no stagnation, which can cause health problems. Acupuncture treatments, during which the energy meridians are stimulated with needles, are generally designed to move Qi and dispel stagnation.

The liver is also said to "store the soul"; in Chinese medicine the "spirit" is a complex concept combining mental activity, consciousness, determination, animal energies, and Hun, a more ethereal aspect of soul.

Weak knees

The liver is also believed to control the tendons, so joint pains caused by tendon problems are seen as a liver weakness. This is most apparent in the knees. Aching knees the morning after an evening of too much alcohol and rich food are a sure sign that the liver has been working too hard.

Assorted associations

The liver is said to be "seen in the nails" and "linked to the eyes." Again, these attributes are also valuable pointers to the state of the liver: in Western theory pale fingernails can indicate anemia—

a blood deficiency problem that the Chinese associate with the liver. Healthy pink nails suggest good liver Qi. Poor eyesight is also seen as a result of deficient liver blood, while irritant conditions like conjunctivitis are defined in terms of heat or wind affecting the liver.

Gung-ho

In the West we use the term "gung-ho" to describe a sort of excessively jingoistic, military aggression. Theories of the term's derivation vary—one authority suggests it was the name of a Chinese industrial cooperative. Perhaps it is more accurate to say it is a misspelling of Gan Huo ("liver fire") since the liver is also associated with anger and shouting: the archetypal red-faced, short-tempered grouch is a typical manifestation of excess liver fire.

More Information

For more information see: **soul**, pages 212–213; **Huai Niu Xi**, page 111; **menstrual problems**, pages 112–113.

GOU QI ZI Wolfberry

Both wolfberry fruits and root bark (Di Gu Pi) are used in Chinese medicine. The root bark is listed among Shen Nong's "superior woods" as a remedy for "evil Qi," although today the fruits are a more common remedy. A restorative congee (rice porridge) using the berries is a traditional household remedy for kidney Qi deficiency, which is typified by impotence, low back pain, dizziness, and tinnitus.

At A Glance

BOTANICAL NAME
Lycium chinense/L. barbarum

COMMON NAME
Wolfberry, Matrimony vine, Duke of Argyll's tea tree

FAMILY
Solanaceae

PART USED
Fruit

TASTE
Sweet

CHARACTER
Neutral

MERIDIANS
Liver, kidney

ACTIONS
lowers blood pressure, lowers blood sugar levels, liver tonic and restorative, immunostimulant, lowers blood cholesterol levels

TRADITIONAL USES
• to nourish liver and kidney yin
• to nourish the blood
• to brighten the eyes

TYPICAL CHINESE DOSE
¼–½ ounce (6–15 grams)

COMBINATIONS
Used with Wu Wei Zi (schisandra) as an all-purpose tonic for general debility; with Ju Hua (chrysanthemum) for liver deficiency and poor eyesight or eyestrain; and with Dang Gui (Chinese angelica) and Shu Di Huang (Chinese foxglove) for indigestion associated with constrained liver Qi.

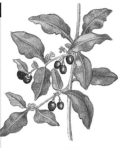

WOLFBERRY

Cautions

Do not use in cases of excess heat and spleen deficiency with dampness.

LONG YAN ROU Longan

Longan fruits are somewhat like raisins and are delicious when added to cakes and rice puddings in cooking, in much the same way as other dried fruits are. Longan fruits have been used in Chinese medicine for at least 2,000 years to combat signs of aging and as a tonic after childbirth. It can also be used to treat insomnia, fatigue, and dizziness. The Chinese name translates as "dragon eye flesh."

At A Glance

BOTANICAL NAME
Dimocarpus longan

COMMON NAME
Longan

FAMILY
Sapindaceae

PART USED
Fruit

TASTE
Sweet

CHARACTER
Warm

MERIDIANS
Heart, spleen

ACTIONS
Nourishing, sedative, antifungal

TRADITIONAL USES
• to tonify heart and spleen and calm the spirit
• to nourish the blood

TYPICAL CHINESE DOSE
¼–⅖ ounce (6–12 grams)

COMBINATIONS
Used with Suan Zao Ren (wild date) for palpitations and insomnia caused by deficient heart blood; with Ren Shen (Korean ginseng), Huang Qi (astragalus), Dang Gui (Chinese angelica), Bai Zhu (white atractylodes), and other herbs in Gui Pi Tang, which is used to replenish Qi and blood and strengthen the heart; and in various combinations for treating insomnia, forgetfulness, dizziness, and fatigue.

LONGAN

Cautions

Avoid in fire and damp phlegm stagnation.

Herbs to Clear Heat

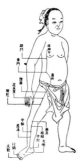

Meridians
Heat can affect all the meridians, resulting in thirst, jaundice, nosebleeds, or skin rashes.

While the six "evils" or external pathogens of wind, heat, cold, dryness, dampness, and fire can initially affect the body's exterior leading to superficial or exterior syndromes, they can also enter the interior if they are left untreated.

Internal heat problems can include many symptoms that we would associate with infections: dysentery, diarrhea, and jaundice, for example, can all be associated with internal heat and dampness, while irritant skin rashes are often blamed on heat entering the blood. Toxic heat invading the blood, for example, can be characterized by nosebleeds, blood in the urine, and spitting or vomiting blood. Conditions that might be given this label include septicemia, acute liver diseases, and severe boils and carbuncles.

Heat can also affect individual acupuncture meridians (channels), the internal organs, and vital energy. Heat affecting the liver channel may be characterized by eye inflammations (since the liver and eye are linked), high blood pressure, and digestive upset. Illnesses that could be blamed on this syndrome include acute conjunctivitis, hepatitis, gallbladder inflammations (cholecystitis), prostatitis, and acute pelvic inflammatory disorders.

Cold, bitter herbs

Herbs for treating this sort of internal heat are always characterized as cold and many are bitter-tasting as well. A typical example is Huang Lian (Chinese gold thread), which is an extremely bitter remedy that can clear heat from the heart, liver, stomach, and large intestine.

Many of these herbs have also been shown to be strongly antibacterial: Lian Qiao (forsythia), for example, is a very effective broad-spectrum antimicrobial. It has been shown to inhibit the growth of bacteria like *Staphylococcus aurea* and *Shigella dysenteriae* (which cause dysentery), *Streptococcus* spp. (often responsible for pneumonia), *Salmonella typhi* (causing typhoid), *Mycobacterium tuberculosis* (which causes TB), and many others.

Other herbs used to combat internal heat problems include: Zhi Mu (*Anemarrhena aspheloides*), Zhi Zi (gardenia), Dan Zhu Ye (*Loptatherum gracile*), Xia Ku Cao (self-heal), Lu Gen (common reed), Lian Zi (lotus seed), and Mi Meng Hua (buddleia).

More Information

Huang Lian, page 138; Lian Zi, page 126; Lian Qiao, page 143; Mi Meng Hua, page 127; Xia Ku Cao, page 123; Zhi Zi, page 122.

ZHI ZI Gardenia

The fruits of the gardenia plant are an important remedy for quelling fire in high fevers, inflamed eyes, or acute hepatitis. Zhi Zi have been used to clear hot conditions since the days of Shen Nong, who recommended it for treating "evil Qi in the five internal [organs]" as well as "drinker's nose." The herb is used raw to combat heat and dampness and can be stir-fried for heat in the blood or carbonized to improve its styptic (stops external bleeding) action.

At A Glance

BOTANICAL NAME
Gardenia jasminoides

COMMON NAME
Gardenia

FAMILY
Rubiaceae

PART USED
Fruit

TASTE
Bitter

CHARACTER
Cold

MERIDIANS
Heart, lung, liver, gallbladder, stomach, San Jiao

ACTIONS
Antibacterial, antifungal, antiparasitic, stimulates bile flow, lowers blood pressure, laxative, sedative

TRADITIONAL USES
• to clear heat and relieve irritability
• to drain damp heat
• to clear heat and fire poisons from the blood

TYPICAL CHINESE DOSE
1/10–1/3 ounce (3–10 grams)

COMBINATIONS
Used with Mu Dan Pi (tree peony) for problems such a period pain and headaches linked to heat caused by deficient liver blood; with Sheng Di Huang (Chinese foxglove) and other herbs for hemorrhage caused by heat, such as nosebleeds; and with Hua Shi (talcum) for damp heat in the bladder causing conditions such as cystitis.

GARDENIA

Cautions

Avoid if diarrhea is present.

XIA KU CAO

Self-heal This is a common European wildflower, traditionally used in folk medicine as an herb for healing wounds—hence its common name. The Chinese name literally means "summer dry herb" and the plant was listed by Shen Nong as a remedy for heat problems including "swollen feet." It as an important cooling remedy for the liver and it can be very effective at calming hyperactive children who are suffering from liver fire syndromes.

At A Glance

BOTANICAL NAME
Prunella vulgaris

COMMON NAME
Self-heal

FAMILY
Labiatae/Lamiaceae

PART USED
Flower spike

TASTE
Bitter, pungent

CHARACTER
Cool

MERIDIANS
Lung, gallbladder

ACTIONS
Antibacterial, lowers blood pressure, stimulates urine flow, astringent, and wound herb

TRADITIONAL USES
• to clear heat from the liver
• to dissipate nodules

TYPICAL CHINESE DOSE
¼–⅓ ounce (6–10 grams)

COMBINATIONS
Used with Ju Hua (chrysanthemum) for headaches and dizziness linked to ascending liver fire; with Xiang Fu (nutgrass) for eye pains; or with Dang Gui (Chinese angelica) and Bai Shao Yao (white peony) for eye pain associated with deficient liver Qi. It is also used with Chai Hu (bupleurum) for constrained liver Qi that is characterized by the swelling of the lymph nodes.

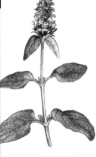

SELF-HEAL

Cautions

Avoid if the spleen or stomach are weak.

Interior Syndromes

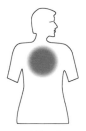

Qi level

As external heat moves to the interior, it can affect particular organs, such as the lungs or spleen, at the Qi stage before moving on to affect the blood (Xue).

While external or superficial problems are usually minor and self-limiting, illnesses related to an internal problem are regarded as much more serious.

As well as problems associated with external pathogens moving into the interior, usually because of inadequate or inappropriate treatment, Chinese medicine has two other explanations for how an interior syndrome can develop. Either the internal organs might be invaded directly by the external pathogens—such as "interior cold" caused by eating too much cold or raw food, or the organs may be affected by emotional disturbances leading to deficient functionality. There are an enormous number of interior syndromes, each with a set of symptoms that can be difficult to translate neatly into a conventional Western disease label.

Pattern of four stages

In 1798 a Chinese physician, Ye Tian-shi, introduced the theory of Wei, Qi, Ying, and Xue to TCM. This is a method for identifying symptom-complexes that are caused by external heat evils moving through different parts of the system, starting with the Wei Qi, or superficial defense energy.

Known as the "pattern of four stages" (Wei Qi Ying Xue Bian Zheng), the approach tracks a heat attack as it moves from the superficial Wei stage, through to the Qi level that affects particular organs, which is then followed by an attack on Ying or the nutritive Qi, and finally by an attack on the blood (Xue) itself.

Internal heat syndromes

As invading external heat moves inwardly through the system, following the four-stage pattern, it creates different groups of symptoms and disharmonies, affecting different organs. At the Qi level there may be heat affecting the lungs with coughing and breathing problems, or there could be heat building up in the intestines leading to constipation and abdominal distension. These different organ syndromes are also always accompanied by fever, thirst, and fidgeting or restlessness.

At the Ying level heat can affect body fluids to cause dry mouth, night fevers, insomnia, or faint skin rashes, while at the Xue level there can be nosebleeds, blood in the stools, coughing or vomiting blood, and skin rashes.

More Information

For more information see **Wei Qi**, page 84; **Xue**, pages 96–97; **Ying Qi**, page 88.

LIAN Lotus

The lotus is one of the East's most sacred plants. It is associated in India with the dawning of spiritual awareness and so it is often used for offerings in temples. The lotus has been used medicinally since ancient Egyptian times and almost all its parts are used in China for a wide range of ailments, including insomnia, fever, dysentery, and palpitations.

At A Glance

BOTANICAL NAME
Nelumbo nucifera

COMMON NAME
Lotus

FAMILY
Nymphaeaceae

PARTS USED
Seed (Lian Zi); stamens (Lian Xu); flower stem (Lian Fang); seed plumule/radicle (Lian Zi Xin); root (Ou Jie); leaves (He Je)

TASTE
Sweet, astringent; flower stems: bitter, astringent; leaves: bitter

CHARACTER
Mostly cooling or neutral

MERIDIANS
Heart, spleen, kidney

ACTIONS
Aphrodisiac, astringent, stops bleeding, tonic, nervine

TRADITIONAL USES
Lian Zi: • tonifies the spleen and stops diarrhea/tonifies kidney energy/calming. Ou Jie: • clears stagnant blood/stops bleeding/removes heat from blood. Lian Zi Xin: • quells heart fire

TYPICAL CHINESE DOSE
Ou Jie: ⅓–1 ounce (9–30 grams); Lian Zi: ⅓–⅗ ounce (9–18 grams) ; Lian Zi Xin: ⁷⁄₁₀₀–¼ ounce (2–6 grams)

COMBINATIONS
Lian Zi is used with Huang Lian (Chinese gold thread) and Dang Shen (asiabell root) for dysentery, insomnia, and palpitations linked to heart/kidney dysfunction. Lian Zi Xin with Xuan Shen (ningpo figwort) and Mai Men Dong (lilyturf) for high fevers. Ou Jie with Chuan Bei Mu (tendrilled fritillary) and Sheng Di Huang (Chinese fox-glove) for heat in the lungs.

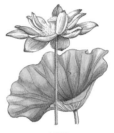

LOTUS

Cautions

Avoid if constipated.

MI MENG HUA Buddleia

Introduced to Europe by the nineteenth-century plant hunters, buddleia has become a common weed in many areas and it has colonized railroad embankments and quarries. The herb affects the liver meridian and is mostly used for eye problems. Its use dates back to the Song Dynasty in the tenth century.

At A Glance

BOTANICAL NAME
Buddleia officinalis

COMMON NAME
Buddleia

FAMILY
Loganiaceae/Buddleiaceae

PART USED
Flower

TASTE
Sweet

CHARACTER
Cool

MERIDIANS
Liver

ACTIONS
Antispasmodic, mild diuretic (stimulates urine flow)

TRADITIONAL USES
• to clear heat in the liver
• to benefit the eyes

TYPICAL CHINESE DOSE
⅒–⅓ ounce (3–9 grams)

COMBINATIONS
Mi Meng Hua is used with Gou Qi Zi (wolfberry fruits) and other herbs for blurred vision, poor eyesight, or cataracts that are associated with deficient liver and kidney energy.

BUDDLEIA

Cautions

None known

Eczema

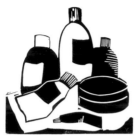

Orthodox view
Western medicine usually treats eczema with an assortment of creams, ointments, and internal medicines.

In the West most skin problems, including eczema, tend to be treated by orthodox practitioners in much the same way, usually with anti-inflammatory creams. Western herbalists will generally include herbs in their remedy order to stimulate the circulation and liver to help clear any toxins that are contributing to the problem. Chinese medicine also sees eczema as part of wider disharmony within the system, so it is important to identify this underlying cause when deciding on the remedy.

Heat invading the blood is a common cause, but eczema can also be due to an attack by superficial cold-wind-damp, heat-damp, or be related to lung problems since the lungs and skin are closely linked in the five element model. This is one reason why standardized over-the-counter eczema remedies based on traditional Chinese prescriptions are not always effective—they may be treating the wrong cause.

A well-publicized eczema program at Great Ormond Street Hospital for children in London was carried out during the 1990s. A semistandardized formula was used, aimed at treating the sort of eczema caused by external heat invading the blood—usually the chronic, dry, red, irritant variety. The remedy included:

• **Chi Shao Yao** (red peony)—cooling to remove heat from the blood;

• **Mu Dan Pi** (tree peony)—cools blood and improves blood circulation;

• **Sheng Di Huang** (Chinese foxglove)—cooling to clear heat and nourish blood and yin;

• **Dan Zhu Ye** (*Loptatherum gracile*)—clears heat and reduces irritation;

• **Fang Feng** (ledebouriella)—a slightly warming herb used to clear superficial wind (both wind-cold and wind-heat) and dampness. It is also used for irritant skin disorders associated with wind/damp problems;

• **Bai Xian Pi** (dittany bark)—clears heat, fire poisons, and wind-damp;

• **Mu Tong** (chocolate vine)—cold, bitter, and anti-inflammatory;

• **Zi Hua Di Ding** (Yoedons violets) an anti-inflammatory—clears heat and toxins;

• **Ci Ji Li** (*Tribulis terrestris*)—an energizing liver yang remedy.

In the trial more than 50 percent of eczema sufferers showed improvements after four weeks of treatment. However, 10 percent of those involved dropped out of the trial; they could not bear the taste of the Chinese decoction.

More Information

For more information see: **Chi Shao Yao**, page 110; **Mu Dan Pi**, page 134; **Sheng Di Huang**, page 130.

DI HUANG Chinese foxglove

Di Huang is used raw (Sheng Di Huang), stir-fried with wine (Shu Di Huang), or occasionally cooked without wine (Gan Di Huang). Sheng Di Huang, is cold, used to clear heat, and is more helpful for yin and body fluids, while Shu Di Huang is a major blood tonic used for menstrual problems. Shen Nong suggested that regular use could prevent senility.

At A Glance

BOTANICAL NAME
Rehmannia glutinosa

COMMON NAME
Chinese foxglove

FAMILY
Scrophulariaceae

PART USED
Tuberous root

TASTE
Sweet; Sheng Di Huang is also bitter

CHARACTER
Shu Di Huang—slightly warm
Sheng Di Huang—cold

MERIDIANS
Heart, liver, kidney

ACTIONS
Improves heart function, stimulates urine flow, mild laxative, reduces blood sugar

TRADITIONAL USES
Shu Di Huang:
• to nourish blood and regulate menstrual flow
• to replenish kidney yin
Sheng Di Huang:
• to clear heat
• to nourish yin and promote body fluids

TYPICAL CHINESE DOSE
⅓–1 ounce (9–30 grams)

COMBINATIONS
Sheng Di Huang is used with Xuan Shen (ningpo figwort) for fire syndromes and fevers; with Bai Shao Yao (white peony) for heat symptoms linked to deficient blood. Shu Di Huang with Shan Zhu Yu (dogwood) and Shan Yao (Chinese yam) for dizziness and back pains linked to deficient liver and kidneys; and with Suan Zao Ren (wild date) for insomnia and palpitations.

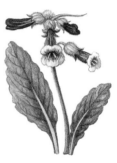

CHINESE FOXGLOVE

Cautions

Not to be used with diarrhea, poor appetite, or indigestion.

XUAN SHEN Ningpo figwort

Xuan Shen was also included in Shen Nong's herbal and is an extremely effective herb for clearing fire poisons. Shen Nong includes it in the "middle class" and suggests that it can strengthen kidney Qi and brighten the eyes. He also recommended it for problems like mastitis in breastfeeding. The Chinese name translates as "dark root."

At A Glance

BOTANICAL NAME
Scrophularia ningpoensis

COMMON NAME
Ningpo figwort

FAMILY
Scrophulariaceae

PART USED
Root

TASTE
Bitter, salty

CHARACTER
Cold

MERIDIANS
lung, stomach, kidney

ACTIONS
Antibacterial, antiviral, improves heart function, lowers blood pressure, lowers blood sugar levels

TRADITIONAL USES
• to nourish yin and Jing
• to clear heat and fire poisons
• to soften and dissipate hard swellings and nodules

TYPICAL CHINESE DOSE
⅓–1 ounce (9–30 grams)

COMBINATIONS
Xuan Shen is used with Mu Dan Pi (tree peony) for skin rashes; with Niu Bang Zi (burdock) for acute sore throats associated with wind-heat; with Lian Qiao (forsythia) for deep-seated dental abscesses, and with Xia Ku Cao (self-heal) and Zhe Bei Mu (fritillary) for swellings, throat problems, and goiter often associated with phlegm.

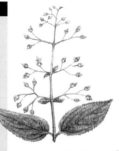

NINGPO FIGWORT

Cautions

Avoid if diarrhea is present.

The Seven Emotions

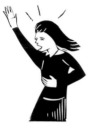

Joy

Joy is associated with the heart and represents a more manic or overexcited aspect of joy than our usual Western interpretation.

The "seven emotions" can also be the cause of interior illnesses. If these emotions become excessive or persistent, they may lead to imbalance and illness will follow.

Joy

This emotion is linked to the heart and to the Western mind it is a cheerful, positive emotion that we find difficult to see as damaging. The negative side of joy can be manic or inappropriate behavior that will damage the heart and lungs, which are located close by in the upper Jiao. Excess joy damaging heart Qi can lead to an inability to concentrate, while hysterical laughter within some mental disorders is associated by the Chinese with damaged heart Qi.

Fright

Panic or sudden fear from some dramatic event is also associated with the heart—an association that we can easily understand in the West from the symptoms of "panic attacks" with their palpitations, mental restlessness, and cold sweats. In Chinese medicine the fright is said to send the heart Qi "wandering about adhering to nothing."

Worry

Worry is the emotion linked to the spleen. Dwelling too much on a problem or concentrating for too long and too hard can lead to stagnation of spleen Qi, which is presented as depression, anxiety, poor appetite, weakened limbs, abdominal bloating, and menstrual irregularities.

Sadness

Sadness is linked to the lungs and an excess is said to "consume lung Qi," leading to respiratory problems. Bronchitis and asthmatic problems often seem to follow bereavement, while chest coughs are common in those who are unhappy.

Grief

Extreme grief or shock is also linked to the lungs and, since the lungs are responsible for the entire Qi circulation, severe shock affects the entire body.

Fear

Fear is linked to the kidney and an excess will reverse the normal, upward flow of kidney Qi leading to listlessness, lower back pains, urinary problems, and a desire for solitude.

Anger

In TCM the liver is associated with anger, too much causes the liver Qi to rise, which leads to headaches, a flushed face, dizziness, and red eyes.

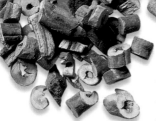

MU DAN PI Tree peony

The tree peony—another garden ornamental in the West—is an important herb for cooling blood. It was first listed in a twelfth-century Chinese herbal known as the "Pouch of Pearls" (*Zhen Zhu Nang*). The raw root is preferred to treat heat in the blood but is stir-fried in cases of blood stagnation or roasted and carbonized to stop bleeding.

At A Glance

BOTANICAL NAME
Paeonia suffruticosa

COMMON NAME
Tree peony, mountain peony

FAMILY
Paeoniacea

PART USED
Root bark

TASTE
Bitter, pungent

CHARACTER
Slightly cold

MERIDIANS
Heart, liver, kidney

ACTIONS
Antibacterial, antiallergenic, anti-inflammatory, analgesic, lowers blood pressure, sedative

TRADITIONAL USES
• to clear heat and cool blood
• to invigorate blood and clear blood stagnation
• to clear ascending liver fire

TYPICAL CHINESE DOSE
¼–²⁄₅ ounce (6–12 grams)

COMBINATIONS
Used with Chi Shao Yao (red peony) for skin rashes, blood in the sputum, or vomit associated with heat in the blood; with Sheng Di Huang (Chinese foxglove) and other herbs for fevers associated with heat; with Gui Zhi (cinnamon twigs) for chest pains linked to stagnant blood syndromes; with Ju Hua (chrysanthemum) for ascending liver fire; and with Jin Yin Hua (honeysuckle) and Lian Qiao (forsythia) for boils, carbuncles, and similar inflammations associated with fire poisons.

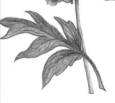

TREE PEONY

Cautions

Avoid in pregnancy or diarrhea.

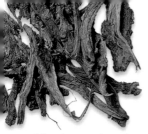

HUANG QIN Baical

skullcap Western varieties of skullcap are classified as nervines or sedatives, but the Chinese member of the family is primarily used for clearing damp heat—both external and internal. The plant was included in Shen Nong's herbal in the "middle class" of herbal remedies as a remedy for diarrhea, dysentery, and jaundice.

At A Glance

BOTANICAL NAME
Scutellaria baicalensis

COMMON NAME
Baical skullcap

FAMILY
Labiatae/Lamiaceae

PART USED
Root

TASTE
Bitter

CHARACTER
Cold

MERIDIANS
Lung, heart, stomach, gallbladder, large intestines

ACTIONS
Antibacterial, antispasmodic, stimulates urine flow, reduces fever, lowers blood cholesterol

TRADITIONAL USES
• to clear heat and quell fire
• to drain damp heat
• to calm the fetus (in threatened miscarriage)
• to eliminate heat in the lung and calm liver yang

TYPICAL CHINESE DOSE
⅒–⅓ ounce (3–9 grams)

COMBINATIONS
Used with other cooling herbs like Huang Lian (Chinese gold thread) for feverish chills with symptoms of thick yellow sputum, thirst, and irritability. Used with Bai Shao Yao (white peony), Zhi Zi (gardenia), Huang Bai (amur cork tree), Mu Dan Pi (tree peony), or Da Huang (Chinese rhubarb) for damp-heat problems linked to dysentery, nosebleeds, or vomiting blood.

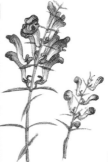

BAICAL SKULLCAP

Cautions

If a person is without true heat and dampness symptoms.

Internal Damp-heat Problems

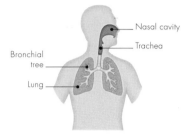

Bronchial tree
Lung
Nasal cavity
Trachea

Wind-heat

Invasion of the lungs by wind-heat can be similar to acute bronchitis or a severe chest cold in the West.

External pathogens often act in combination to cause superficial syndromes—they also do this when they invade the interior. Treatment is usually a combination of the herbs used to combat the particular "evils" with other remedies to focus on specific areas.

Wind-heat invading the lung

Wind-heat invading the lung would be characterized by the same symptoms as wind-heat in the exterior—fever, skin eruption, dry mouth, and thirst—but with an additional cough and thick yellow sputum. In the West we might label this as acute bronchitis. A typical Chinese remedy is Sang Ju Yin, which includes:

- **Sang Ye** (mulberry leaves)—to clear wind-heat;
- **Ju Hua** (chrysanthemum)—to clear wind-heat;
- **Xing Ren** (apricot seeds)—an antitussive (relieves coughs) and antiasthmatic remedy;
- **Jie Geng** (balloon flower)—helps to clear phlegm and soothe the lung;
- **Bo He** (field mint)—a wind-heat remedy;
- **Lian Qiao** (forsythia)—clears heat and toxins from the blood;
- **Lu Gen** (common reed)—a cooling remedy to reduce fevers; and
- **Gan Cao** (licorice root)—to harmonize the mixture.

If the sputum was profuse then the physician might add Zhe Bei Mu (fritillary) to the mix as well to help resolve phlegm.

Summer diarrhea

What the West would label as acute gastroenteritis is seen in TCM as being caused by either damp-cold or damp-heat. The damp-cold variety is typified by watery diarrhea and thin vomit with a preference for hot, soothing drinks, while the damp-heat sort is likely to be accompanied by thirst, fever, a burning sensation in the lower bowel, and foul-smelling stools. Summer diarrhea —common in hot weather and usually blamed on food poisoning—is often a damp-heat problem.

Cold, bitter herbs are used for the damp-heat variety to clear the invading pathogens, while aromatic herbs may be added to normalize spleen and stomach function. A common remedy is Ge Gen Huang Qin Huang Lian Tang. This is a decoction combining Ge Gen (kudzu root), Huang Lian (Chinese gold thread), and Huang Qin (baical skullcap) with a little Gan Cao (licorice root) to help to harmonize the mixture.

HUANG LIAN Chinese gold thread

Huang Lian has been used as a bitter, cold remedy to clear heat and damp for at least 2,000 years. Shen Nong referred to it as Wang Lian (King lily) and listed the plant among the "superior" herbs, suggesting that regular use of the plant would also improve the memory. Its Chinese name translates as "yellow links" and it is one of an important group of cooling "yellow" herbs.

At A Glance

BOTANICAL NAME
Coptis chinensis

COMMON NAME
Chinese gold thread

FAMILY
Ranunculaceae

PARTS USED
Root and rhizome

TASTE
Bitter

CHARACTER
Cold

MERIDIANS
Heart, liver, stomach, large intestine

ACTIONS
Antibacterial, lowers blood pressure, stimulates acetylcholine production, sedative, anti-inflammatory, antifungal, stimulates bile flow

TRADITIONAL USES
• to clear heat, fire, fire poisons, and damp heat
• to calm heart fire
• to drain stomach fire

TYPICAL CHINESE DOSE
³⁄₁₀₀–⁹⁄₅₀ ounce (1–5 grams)

COMBINATIONS
Used with Sheng Di Huang (Chinese foxglove) for heat syndromes causing insomnia, thirst, and delirium; with Wu Zhu Yu (evodia) and Bai Shao Yao (white peony) for abdominal pains, indigestion, dysentery, or stomach upsets; and with Rou Gui (cinnamon bark) for disharmony between heart and kidneys causing insomnia.

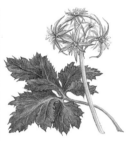

CHINESE GOLD THREAD

Cautions

Avoid if there is diarrhea, yin deficiency (see pages 68–69), or cold deficient stomach. Prolonged use may damage spleen and stomach.

HUANG BAI Amur cork tree

Huang Bai first appears in the Chinese *Materia Medica* in 1578 in the great herbal of Li Shi Zhen—a contemporary of the herbal of John Gerard in England. Huang Bai translates as "yellow fir" and the herb is an important remedy for clearing heat and damp. It is sometimes mixed with salt to nourish yin or with wine to clear heat in the upper Jiao, which is linked to bloodshot eyes and tinnitus.

At A Glance

BOTANICAL NAME
Phellodendron amurense

COMMON NAME
Amur cork tree

FAMILY
Rutaceae

PART USED
Bark

TASTE
Bitter

CHARACTER
Cold

MERIDIANS
Kidney, urinary bladder, large intestine

ACTIONS
Antibacterial, lowers blood pressure, lowers blood sugar, stimulates bile flow, stimulates urine flow

TRADITIONAL USES
• to clear heat and dampness
• to calm fire and detoxify
• to reduce false heat linked to yin deficiency

TYPICAL CHINESE DOSE
1/10–1/3 ounce (3–10 grams)

COMBINATIONS
Used with Chi Shao Yao (red peony) for bleeding and dysentery-like problems, and with Shan Yao (Chinese yam) and Bai Guo (ginkgo seeds) for urinary problems linked to damp-heat.

AMUR CORK TREE

Cautions

Avoid in deficient spleen syndromes, diarrhea, or in those with weak stomachs.

Fire Poisons

"Hot" swellings or "fire poisons" cause inflamed joints

Herbs can help reduce inflammation

Inflammation
Boils, abscesses, and some inflammatory joint disorders can all be linked to fire poisons in TCM.

Among the rather cryptic traditional indications that are given for many Chinese herbs is "clears fire poisons." This is a description that goes back to the days before microbiology when infections and inflammations were blamed on some sort of mysterious poison rather than on bacteria.

Poison (Du) has many meanings in Chinese theory: it can mean pus from boils and carbuncles or it can simply refer to feverish symptoms associated with infectious disease.

A hot, inflamed joint, as is found in some types of arthritis or tendinitis, could be described in TCM as a "hot" (Re) swelling but if the sufferer is also feverish, lethargic, and clearly sick, then it is likely to be called a "hot poison" (Re Du) or "fire poison" (Huo Du) swelling. It is then treated with some of their antipoison remedies.

All sorts of abscesses come into this poison category—from dental abscesses and boils to internal inflammatory problems such as mastitis and appendicitis.

Herbs that are used to treat hot or fire poisons are often anti-inflammatory, antibacterial, antiviral, or antifungal. Although laboratory studies have not proven their effectiveness, many find these to be effective remedies for swelling and infection. Poison herbs are usually categorized as cooling or cold with varying tastes. Depending on the location and the type of poison, herbal remedies can be chosen to target the organ or acupuncture meridian affected.

Herbs for heat and fire poisons

Among the herbs for clearing heat or fire poisons are Jin Yin Hua (honeysuckle), Lian Qiao (forsythia), and Da Qing Ye (woad leaves), the latter being mainly used for conditions like mumps, canker sores, and throat swellings. Ban Lang Gen (woad root) is used in acute fevers.

Severe conditions

Fire poisons were also blamed for critical conditions such as acute appendicitis, which were treated (in the days before surgery) with a cooling mixture of herbs such as Da Huang (Chinese rhubarb), Mu Dan Pi (tree peony), Lian Qiao (forsythia), and Jin Yin Hua (honeysuckle), as well as Zi Hua Di Ding (Yoedons violets) and Pu Gong Ying (Chinese dandelion), classified as specific remedies for "surface suppurations" including boils and mastitis.

More Information

For further information see: **Da Huang**, page 154; **Jin Yin Hua**, page 142; **Lian Qiao**, page 143; **Mu Dan Pi**, page 134.

JIN YIN HUA Honeysuckle

Jin Yin Hua translates from the Chinese as "gold silver flower," which is a good description. This popular white and yellow climber has been familiar in Western gardens since William Kerr collected the first specimens for the Royal Botanical Gardens at Kew, in London, in 1806. The flowers and the stems (Jin Yin Teng) have been used by Chinese practitioners to treat many different heat syndromes since at least the seventh century.

At A Glance

BOTANICAL NAME
Lonicera japonica

COMMON NAME
Honeysuckle

FAMILY
Capriofoliaceae

PART USED
Flowers

TASTE
Sweet

CHARACTER
Cold

MERIDIANS
Lung, stomach, large intestine

ACTIONS
Antibacterial, antiviral, lowers blood pressure.

TRADITIONAL USES
• to clear heat and fire poisons
• to clear damp heat in the lower Jiao in dysentery-like syndromes
• to expel external wind-heat

TYPICAL CHINESE DOSE
1–2 ounces (30–60 grams)

COMBINATIONS
Often used with Lian Qiao (forsythia) as a basic combination for many heat problems: add Huang Qin (baical skullcap) and Huang Lian (Chinese gold thread) for high fevers; Jie Geng (balloon flower) and Niu Bang Zi (burdock) for sore or swollen throats; or Bo He (field mint) for external wind-heat syndromes.

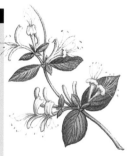

HONEYSUCKLE

Cautions

Avoid in deficient and cold conditions.

LIAN QIAO Forsythia

This plant is familiar in the West as a yellow-flowered garden shrub that was brought to Europe in 1844 by the Scottish explorer Robert Fortune and named after the Scottish botanist William Forsyth. The herb is listed by Shen Nong who recommended it for "malign sores, goiters, and tumors." He gave it the alternative names of Jian Hua (orchid flower) and Yi Qiao (strange beauty).

At A Glance

BOTANICAL NAME
Forsythia suspensa

COMMON NAME
Forsythia

FAMILY
Oleaceae

PART USED
Fruit

TASTE
Bitter

CHARACTER
Slightly cold

MERIDIANS
Lung, heart, gallbladder

ACTIONS
Antibacterial, combats nausea and vomiting, antiparasitic

TRADITIONAL USES
• to clear heat and fire poisons
• to expel wind-heat
• to dissipate nodules and swellings

TYPICAL CHINESE DOSE
¼–½ ounce (6–15 grams)

COMBINATIONS
Often used with Jin Yin Hua (honeysuckle, see left). Also combined with Ju Hua (chrysanthemum) for feverish conditions; with Ma Huang (ephedra), Chi Shao Yao (red peony), and Gan Cao (licorice root) for skin eruptions, including allergic rashes; and with Huang Lian (Chinese gold thread) for acute infections.

FORSYTHIA

Cautions

Avoid in diarrhea associated with deficient spleen, fevers that are linked to deficient Qi (see pages 80–89), and purulent abscesses.

Herbs to Warm the Interior

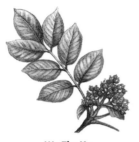

Wu Zhu Yu
Stomach chills could be associated with invasion by interior cold; Wu Zhu Yu (evodia) helps to warm the spleen and stomach.

Just as fire and heat can invade the interior, so, too, can cold. Many interior cold problems are comparatively minor, such as watery diarrhea or abdominal discomfort. Others can be more serious, leading to "devastated yang" or "collapsed Qi," typified by severe shock with icy cold hands and feet, profuse sweating, diarrhea, and collapse.

Interior cold problems are often associated with the spleen and stomach, and many of the herbs classified as warming the interior are actually yang tonics that act primarily on the spleen or kidneys. In Western terms the herbs are usually digestive or circulatory stimulants—some combat nausea and diarrhea while others act as stimulants on the nervous system.

Gan Jiang (dried ginger), for example, is a warm, invigorating remedy that is used for "devastated yang" syndromes as well as for a cold-deficient spleen and stomach. Rou Gui (cinnamon bark) is said to "tonify the fire at the gate of vitality": it is a very hot herb that focuses on the lower Jiao and kidneys.

Other herbs for interior cold include: Fu Zi (prepared aconite), Wu Zhu Yu (evodia), Chuan Jiao (Szechuan or red pepper), Ding Zing (cloves), Xiao Hui Xiang (fennel), Gao Liang Jiang (galangal), Bi Ba (long pepper), and Hu Jiao (black pepper).

The Pattern of Six Stages

Around 220AD the Chinese physician Zhang Zhong-Jie published his classic text *Shang-Han Lun* (or *Discussion of Cold-induced Disorders*). This traces the six stages of a cold-related problem, starting with a superficial attack by external evils and ending with severe internal cold upsetting the yin–yang balance. Zhang's six stages are:

• Tai Yang (greater yang), characterized by fever and headache;

• Yang Ming (yang brightness) with fever, perspiration, and irritability;

• Shao Yang (lesser yang) with alternate chills and fevers, poor appetite, and nausea;

• Tai Yin (greater yin)—cold has moved inside to cause abdominal distension, thirst, vomiting, and diarrhea;

• Shao Yin (lesser yin), characterized by diarrhea, exhaustion, restlessness, cold limbs, and insomnia;

• Jue Yin (absolute yin), characterized by coldness and deficiency syndromes; abdominal pain, nausea, vomiting, cold limbs, and restlessness.

Later critics considered this a gross oversimplification but as a description of how a severe infection could progress in the days before antibiotics it is probably reasonably accurate.

JIANG Ginger

Fresh ginger (Sheng Jiang) is used as a warming remedy for wind-cold chills. Dried ginger (Gan Jiang) has a more tonic action. The peel of fresh ginger root (Sheng Jiang Pi) is used as a diuretic. Shen Nong suggests that long-term use will "enable one to communicate with the spirit." Ginger is widely used in TCM to reduce the toxicity of other herbs.

At A Glance

BOTANICAL NAME
Zingiber officinale

COMMON NAME
Ginger

FAMILY
Zingiberaceae

PART USED
Root

TASTE
Pungent

CHARACTER
Warm

MERIDIANS
Heart, lung, spleen, stomach

ACTIONS
Combats nausea and vomiting, antispasmodic, antiseptic, relieves gas and indigestion, circulatory stimulant, induces sweating, expectorant, relaxes blood vessels, topically: increases blood flow to the skin

TRADITIONAL USES
Sheng Jiang: • releases the exterior, strengthens Wei Qi, and disperses cold
• warms the middle Jiao
• reduces toxicity of other herbs
Gan Jiang: • restores yang
• warms spleen, stomach, and the lung, and resolves phlegm

TRADITIONAL CHINESE DOSE
⅒–⅓ ounce (3–9 grams)

COMBINATIONS
Used with Gan Cao (licorice root) and Gao Liang Jiang (galangal) for cold deficient stomach syndromes; with Bai Zhu (white atractylodes) for deficient spleen; and with Ban Xia (pinellia) and Ren Shen (Korean ginseng) for deficient cold. Sheng Jiang with Ban Xia for vomiting and damp phlegm and with Da Zao (Chinese dates) for external wind-cold.

GINGER

Cautions

Avoid in the various internal heat syndromes.

WU ZHU YU Evodia Wu Zhu

Yu, a toxic herb, has been used as a warming remedy for cold conditions since the days of Shen Nong. He describes it as "warming the center" and dispelling wind, and recommends the root for "killing three kinds of worms." Studies suggest that the fruits can clear pinworms and tapeworms. The plant is mixed with licorice water to reduce its toxicity.

At A Glance

BOTANICAL NAME
Evodia rutaecarpa

COMMON NAME
Evodia

FAMILY
Rutaceae

PART USED
Fruit

TASTE
Pungent, bitter

CHARACTER
Hot, slightly toxic

MERIDIANS
Spleen, stomach, liver, kidney

ACTIONS
Antibacterial, antiparasitic, analgesic, raises body temperature, respiratory stimulant, uterine stimulant

TRADITIONAL USES
• to warm the spleen and stomach
• to dispel cold and relieve pain
• to reverse the flow of Qi

TYPICAL CHINESE DOSE
7/100–1/4 ounce (2–6 grams)

COMBINATIONS
Use with Huang Lian (Chinese gold thread) for vomiting; with Sheng Jiang (fresh ginger) for stomach pain and vomiting; or with Gan Jiang (dried ginger) for cold stomach syndromes and abdominal pain. Also combined with Wu Wei Zi (schisandra) for "cock crow" diarrhea associated with deficient spleen and kidney yang. It is stir-fried to reverse the upward flow of stomach and liver Qi.

EVODIA

Cautions

Avoid in yin deficiency (see pages 68–69) and excess fire.

Cold Syndromes

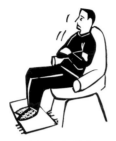

Cold in the limbs
A cold syndrome can be apparent in the way the sufferer looks, walks, and talks: they may be stiff, cramped, and slow.

Cold in the body has a similar effect to cold in the environment. It freezes and congeals, slows down movement, and then leads to underactivity. Cold affecting the channels will therefore block or slow down the circulation of Qi and Xue, leading to sharp cramping pains that are only relieved by hot compresses. Cold in the limbs also causes stiffness and difficulty with movement.

In addition to cold invading the interior, cold conditions can also be associated with imbalances in yin and yang (see pages 68–69 and 72–73). This is because both yang deficiency and yin excess can give the impression of cold.

Digestive problems

Digestive problems accompanied by diarrhea can often be associated with interior cold or yang deficiency. If inner cold is the problem then the condition is likely to be acute and characterized by watery stools, slight fever, and headaches. If yang is deficient then the person also feels cold but this yang deficiency will impair spleen or kidney function. This means that the spleen is unable to transport and transform nutrients and there is a failure of normal water metabolism, which leads to edema or swelling.

In cases of deficient spleen the problem is chronic, and includes frequent bowel movements, poor appetite, and a feeling of oppression and heaviness in the stomach area. Kidney deficiency is typified by "cock crow" diarrhea—a need to rush to the bathroom first thing each morning due to abdominal pains that are then relieved once the visit has been completed.

Each cold problem needs careful diagnosis to ensure appropriate treatment. If interior cold is affecting the body then warming aromatic herbs such as Huo Xiang (patchouli), Bai Zhi (dahurian angelica), and Chen Pi (tangerine peel) are preferred. If spleen deficiency is the problem then a more tonifying mixture with herbs such as Dang Shen (asiabell root), Fu Ling (tuckahoe), Bai Zhu (white atractylodes), and Shan Yao (Chinese yam) would be given. Kidney deficiency needs kidney tonics so the mixture could include Bu Gu Zhi (scurf pea), Wu Zhu Yu (evodia), and Wu Wei Zi (schisandra).

Hot and Cold

"A deficiency of yang brings on exterior cold, while a deficiency of yin leads to interior heat. A preponderance of yang leads to exterior heat, while a preponderance of yin leads to interior cold."

Huang Di Nei Jing Su Wen c. 2500BC

CHUAN JIAO Szechuan pepper

Szechuan peppercorns have been used in TCM since 1350 when they were first listed in the *Household Materia Medica* (*Ri Yong Ben Cao*) by Wu Rui. These peppercorns are unrelated to other types of pepper but are still a popular flavoring in Chinese cooking where they are usually known as Huo Jiao (flower pepper). They look like red peppercorns and are used in spicy dips and as an alternative to five spice powder.

At A Glance

BOTANICAL NAME
Zanthoxylum piperitum var. *bungei*

COMMON NAME
Szechuan pepper, red pepper

FAMILY
Rutaceae

PART USED
Fruit

TASTE
Pungent

CHARACTER
Hot, toxic

MERIDIANS
Spleen, lung, kidney

ACTIONS
Digestive stimulant, antiparasitic, expels intestinal worms, reduces milk flow

TRADITIONAL USES
• to warm the middle Jiao and disperse cold
• to relieve abdominal pain and kill parasites

TYPICAL CHINESE DOSE
$3/100$–$1/10$ ounce (1–3 grams)

COMBINATIONS
Used with Gan Jiang (dried ginger) and Dang Shen (asiabell root) for stomach and abdominal pains and nausea associated with cold deficient stomach and spleen.
Combined with Cang Zhu (gray atractylodes) and Chen Pi (tangerine peel) for cold dampness and diarrhea.

SZECHUAN PEPPER

Cautions

Avoid in deficient yin syndromes (see pages 68–69) with heat symptoms and during pregnancy.

XIAO HUI XIANG

Fennel This herb has been cultivated in Europe since Roman times. The Greeks called the plant *marathron*—reputedly derived from a verb meaning "to grow thin" since it was an early weight-loss aid. In China, it has only been used since the eleventh century. The seeds are considered an important warming remedy for stomach problems and are also believed to affect the liver.

At A Glance

BOTANICAL NAME
Foeniculum vulgare

COMMON NAME
Fennel

FAMILY
Umbelliferae/Apiaceae

PART USED
Seeds

TASTE
Pungent

CHARACTER
Warm

MERIDIANS
Stomach, liver, kidney

ACTIONS
Anti-inflammatory, relieves gas and indigestion, circulatory stimulant, stimulates the flow of milk, stimulates urine flow, mild expectorant

TRADITIONAL USES
• to regulate Qi and alleviate pain
• to warm the stomach and middle Jiao

TYPICAL CHINESE DOSE
1/10–1/3 ounce (3–9 grams)

COMBINATIONS
Used with Rou Gui (cinnamon bark), Sheng Jiang (fresh ginger), or Hou Po (bark of *Magnolia officinalis*) for problems associated with cold in the stomach, including colicky pains, poor appetite, indigestion, and vomiting.

FENNEL

Cautions

Use cautiously in deficient yin syndromes (see pages 68–69).

Downward-draining Herbs

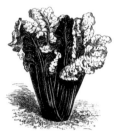

Chinese rhubarb
*Da Huang (Chinese rhubarb) is one
of the most important draining herbs
used in TCM to treat constipation
and other interior excesses.*

Chinese medicine differs, however, in
its explanation of how these remedies
function. All three would, in Western
terms, be described as irritants:
they contain chemicals called
anthraquinone glycosides, which
irritate the gut lining to stimulate
peristalsis—the gut motions that force
the remains of the food we eat through
the colon to be excreted.

In Chinese theory these strong
laxatives are described as clearing
some sort of interior excess—an
overabundance of either heat or
cold that is upsetting the system and
therefore causing constipation.

The group also contains remedies
that are termed "moist laxatives," and
these are usually nuts or seeds that
lubricate the intestine to combat the
dryness or the lack of body fluids
that can also cause constipation.
The group includes Huo Ma Ren
(cannabis seeds) and Yu Li Ren (a type
of cherry seed). This sort of problem
is frequently associated with yin
deficiency and debility.

Downward-draining herbs are
mainly used to stimulate and
lubricate the digestive tract
to improve function and combat
constipation. In Western terms they
would be labeled laxative or purgative
and many are plants that are very
familiar in the West.

Da Huang (Rhubarb root), Lu Hui
(bitter aloes), and Fan Xie Ye (senna
leaf) are all plants that are used by
Western herbalists and orthodox
practitioners for constipation.

Potent cathartics

Chinese medicine also includes a group of very violent cathartics that will induce diarrhea. These are used in severe illness when constipation is linked to stagnation of internal fluids: conditions such as pleurisy or severe edema would be categorized as interior excess syndromes and treated with these strong remedies.

These remedies are not for home use. They are extremely potent and can easily damage yin and body fluids by their overactivity. The group includes Qian Niu Zi (morning glory seeds), Da Ji (Peking spurge), Shang Lu (oriental poke root), Yuan Hua (Daphne flowers), and Gan Sui (oriental spurge).

Laxative Remedies

Chinese laxative remedies are classified as purgatives (e.g. Da Huang, Chinese rhubarb), moist laxatives (e.g., Huo Ma Ren—cannabis seeds), and harsh expellants (cathartics; e.g Qian Niu Zi, morning glory seeds).

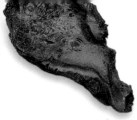

DA HUANG Chinese rhubarb

Da Huang literally means "big yellow" in Chinese because of the color of its root. It is used mainly as a purgative, much as it is in traditional Western herbal treatments. The plant was first brought to Europe by Arab traders and was erroneously thought to originate in the Middle East, hence its common name of Turkey rhubarb.

At A Glance

BOTANICAL NAME
Rheum palmatum

COMMON NAME
Chinese rhubarb,
Turkey rhubarb

FAMILY
Polygonaceae

PARTS USED
Root and rhizome

TASTE
Bitter

CHARACTER
Cold

MERIDIANS
Liver, spleen, stomach,
large intestine

ACTIONS
Purgative, antibacterial,
antifungal, antiparasitic, lowers
blood pressure, lowers blood
cholesterol levels, stimulates bile
flow, stimulates urine flow, and
stops or reduces bleeding

TRADITIONAL USES
• to drain heat including
damp-heat and excess heat
in the blood
• to invigorate blood circulation
and clear blood stagnation
• to detoxify fire poisons

TYPICAL CHINESE DOSE
⅒–⅖ ounce (3–12 grams)

COMBINATIONS
Used with Huang Lian (Chinese
gold thread) and Huang Bai
(amur cork tree) for abdominal
distension and vomiting due to
excess heat or heat in the
blood; with Rou Gui (cinnamon
bark) for chronic constipation;
with Ren Shen (Korean
ginseng) and Gan Jiang (dried
ginger) for diarrhea or
constipation associated with
spleen yang deficiency; and
with Zhi Zi (gardenia), Chai
Hu (bupleurum), and Huang
Bai (amur cork tree) for internal
heat and damp syndromes.

CHINESE RHUBARB

Cautions

Avoid in cases where there
are no heat or fire symptoms;
avoid in pregnancy.

154

HUO MA REN Cannabis

Although regarded as an illegal drug, marijuana is an important medicinal plant. In many areas it is legal by prescription and used in conjunction with other treatments for a variety of medical conditions including glaucoma, multiple sclerosis, and cancer. In China the seeds are used as a laxative.

At A Glance

BOTANICAL NAME
Cannabis sativa

COMMON NAME
Cannabis, hemp, marijuana

FAMILY
Cannibiaceae

PART USED
Seeds

TASTE
Sweet

CHARACTER
Neutral

MERIDIANS
Spleen, stomach, large intestine

ACTIONS
Laxative, lowers blood pressure

TRADITIONAL USES
• to lubricate the intestines
• to nourish yin
• to clear heat and heal sores

TYPICAL CHINESE DOSE
⅓–1 ounce (9–30 grams)

COMBINATIONS
Used with Dang Gui (Chinese angelica) for treating constipation in the elderly or after childbirth that is often related to lack of energy and fluids. The seeds are often supplied in Ma Zi Ren Wan (cannabis seed pills, see page 157), which is named after the plant's alternative Chinese name, Ma Zi Ren.

It is illegal to grow, possess, or use cannabis plants in the US. Herb suppliers sell boiled cannabis seeds so that they cannot be cultivated.

CANNABIS

Cautions

Not to be used if diarrhea is present.

Constipation

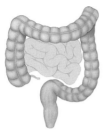

Large intestine

In TCM disorders of the intestine, such as constipation, can have different causes and are diagnosed carefully.

In Chinese theory constipation is a problem associated with the large intestine. In the five element model, the large intestine is the hollow (Fu) organ linked to the lung. In TCM, lung weaknesses can occasionally be associated with constipation.

It is more likely, however, that the problem is associated with a digestive problem due to spleen disharmonies and fluid metabolism.

TCM details five different sorts of constipation, which are due to:

- excess internal heat;
- excess internal cold;
- weakness and debility, as in the elderly or following childbirth;
- dry-heat syndromes with insufficiency of body fluids affecting the digestive tract so making the motion of stools difficult;
- kidney and spleen weakness.

Correct diagnosis is important because if the problem is weakness and debility then strong purgative herbs would be inappropriate. And, as internal heat and cold are possible causes, differentiating between the two is important: excess heat is often associated with a mixed pattern of constipation or loose stools and may have been preceded by fever, skin irritations, and thirst. Constipation associated with excess cold will probably be accompanied by abdominal pain and distension. Da Huang (Chinese rhubarb) is used for both types, with additional remedies helping to make the overall prescription rather more cooling or heating as needed. A cold purgative mix, for example, could include Mu Dan Pi (tree peony), which is slightly cold, with Tao Ren (peach seeds) that are neutral in character. A warming brew would combine Da Huang (Chinese rhubarb) with Sheng Jiang (fresh ginger). For constipation due to energy weakness, tonic herbs are needed—Dang Gui (Chinese angelica), for example. Problems with yin deficiency need cooling remedies such as Ze Xie (water plantain).

Ma Zi Ren Wan

A typical combination for constipation associated with dry heat in the stomach and intestines and insufficiency of body fluids is Ma Zi Ren Wan (cannabis seed pills). These are made from:

Huo Ma Ren	1 ounce (30 grams)
Bai Shao Yao	½ ounce (15 grams)
Xing Ren	⅓ ounce (9 grams)
Zhi Shi	⅓ ounce (9 grams)
Da Huang	⅓ ounce (9 grams)
Hou Po	⅓ ounce (9 grams)

The powdered herbs are usually made into tiny pills produced by mixing them with honey or a similar binding agent, and compressing them together. They are then supplied in bottles with a recommended dose of 10–20 pills in water 2–3 times daily.

FAN XIE YE

Senna The leaves and pods of the senna plant have been used for centuries in many parts of the world as a potent laxative. Today the herb still features in orthodox medicine and can be found in numerous over-the-counter remedies. Senna works by irritating the digestive tract and so encouraging peristalsis. The pods are somewhat milder in action than the leaves, though in Chinese medicine it is only the leaves that are used.

At A Glance

BOTANICAL NAME
Senna alexandrina

COMMON NAME
Senna

FAMILY
Leguminosae/
Caesalpiniaceae

PART USED
Leaves

TASTE
Sweet, bitter

CHARACTER
Cold

MERIDIANS
Large intestine

ACTIONS
Stimulating laxative, antibacterial, expels parasitic worms, cooling

TRADITIONAL USES
• to clear excessive heat from the body
• to drain downward and move stools

TYPICAL CHINESE DOSE
⅒–¼ ounce (3–6 grams)

COMBINATIONS
Usually given individually as a tea or in powder.

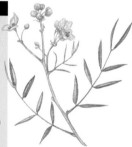

SENNA

Cautions

Avoid in pregnancy; overdose can cause nausea and abdominal pain.

LU HUI **Aloe**

Extracts of aloe vera are used in the West externally for soothing burns and skin sores while internally the plant is increasingly marketed as a tonic remedy. It is strongly purgative (it was once known as "bitter aloes") and is sometimes used for constipation. In China it has been used as a draining remedy since the eleventh century, first appearing in the *Jia You Ben Cao* (*Materia Medica of the Jia You Era*) by Zhang Yu-Xi and Su Song.

At A Glance

BOTANICAL NAME
Aloe vera

COMMON NAME
Aloe

FAMILY
Liliaceae/Aloaceae

PARTS USED
Leaf juice

TASTE
Bitter

CHARACTER
Cold

MERIDIANS
Liver, stomach, large intestine

ACTIONS
Purgative, stimulates bile flow, wound healer, tonic, demulcent, antifungal, stops external bleeding, sedative, expels parasitic worms

TRADITIONAL USES
• to purge heat and fire in the liver and large intestine
• to move stools
• to strengthen the stomach

TYPICAL CHINESE DOSE
3/100–7/100 ounce (1–2 grams)

COMBINATIONS
Lu Hui is used with herbs like Huang Qin (baical skullcap) and Long Dan Cao (Japanese gentian) for excess heat in the liver channel associated with abdominal pain and headaches

ALOE

Cautions

Avoid in pregnancy and in cold deficient spleen or stomach syndromes.

Herbs to Clear Painful Obstructions

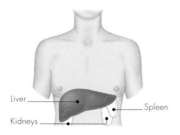

Zang-organ tonics
TCM often uses Zang-organ tonics to treat obstructions related to their associated tissues.

Liver

Kidneys

Spleen

External pathogens moving inside and affecting the interior can cause painful obstructions in the meridians, which in turn lead to pain and distension. If the limb meridians are afflicted then Bì syndrome (Bì Zheng) is the result. Bì is usually translated in the West as "pain" and Bì Zheng as "painful obstructions." Although the term can refer to any disease that is associated with a type of obstruction, Bì syndrome is usually taken to mean diseases that in the West would be classified as arthritis or rheumatic disorders.

Herbs to clear wind-damp

With a variety of different "evils" involved, herbs to treat painful obstructions can include cooling, drying, and warming remedies and the combination is selected to match the specific syndrome, age, and constitution of the patient as well as the particular stage of the illness at the time of treatment.

Many of the herbs used for arthritic problems are tonics for the liver or kidney, which are used to strengthen their associated tissues from the five element model. For example, the liver is linked to tendons while the kidneys are associated with bones. For the muscular aches and pains of rheumatism, spleen tonics would be used instead since the spleen is closely associated with muscles.

Herbs in this group would usually be described in the West as anti-inflammatory or analgesic.

Hu Gu (tiger bones) are one of the more controversial remedies of Chinese medicine, rightly condemned in the West for the threat it poses to the survival of tigers in the wild. They are now known to be highly anti-inflammatory and to combat experimentally-induced arthritis in laboratory animals, which accounts for their persistent use and popularity in many parts of Asia.

All Sorts of Names

Chinese terms can be difficult to transliterate into English letters because the same spelling can indicate several different words depending on how the term is pronounced. There are least three ways of pronouncing every word depending on where in the mouth the tongue is placed at the time. Bi can indicate "painful obstructions" but Bi with a slightly different pronunciation can also mean "retention of urine," while the third pronunciation means "thigh." Adding to the confusion is Bi, "nose"— Bi Sai is used to describe a "stuffy nose."

DU HUO
Pubescent angelica

Du Huo was listed by Shen Nong as a remedy for treating wind-cold as well as relieving pain, epilepsy, and tetanus. He also suggested that long-term use could "slow aging" and gave it the alternative names of Qiang Qing (Qiang green-blue) and Qiang Huo (Qiang activator). The Qiang were a nomadic tribe living in northernwestern China. Nowadays Qiang Huo is the name given to *Notopterygium incisium*, another wind-cold-damp remedy.

Datafile

BOTANICAL NAME
Angelica pubescens

COMMON NAME
Pubescent angelica

FAMILY
Umbelliferae/Apiaceae

PART USED
Root

TASTE
Pungent, bitter

CHARACTER
Slightly warm

MERIDIANS
Kidney, urinary bladder

ACTIONS
Analgesic, antirheumatic, lowers blood pressure, nervous stimulant

TRADITIONAL USES
• to dispel wind and damp
• to relieve pain

TYPICAL CHINESE DOSE
¹⁄₁₀–¹⁄₃ ounce (3–9 grams)

COMBINATIONS
Used in Du Huo Ju Sheng Tang, a mixture of 15 herbs including Du Zhong (eucommia), Rou Gui (cinnamon bark), Dang Gui (Chinese angelica), and Bai Shao Yao (white peony). This remedy is used for chronic lumbago associated with wind-cold-damp and liver or kidney weakness. Du Hao is also combined with Ma Huang (ephedra) for external wind-cold problems; and with Bai Zhu (white atractylodes) for toothaches due to wind-cold.

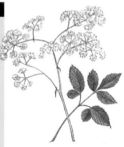

PUBESCENT ANGELICA

Cautions

Avoid in deficient yin (see pages 68–69) and deficient blood syndromes.

SANG Mulberry

The mulberry is one of China's most versatile medicinal trees because the leaves (Sang Ye), root bark (Sang Bai Pi), fruit spikes (Sang Shen), and twigs (Sang Zhi) are all used in slightly different ways. Mulberry leaves were included in Shen Nong's herbal while the other parts of the plant were added in at a later date. The berries, leaves, and bark of a related species (black mulberry, *Morus nigra*) have all been used in Western medicine.

At A Glance

BOTANICAL NAME
Morus alba

COMMON NAME
Mulberry

FAMILY
Moraceae

PARTS USED
Leaves, twigs, root bark, fruit spikes

TASTE
Sweet or bitter

CHARACTER
Cold or neutral

MERIDIANS
Lung, liver, spleen, heart

ACTIONS
Analgesic, antiasthmatic, antibacterial, relieves coughs, induces sweating, stimulates urine flow, expectorant

TRADITIONAL USES
Sang Ye: • clears wind and heat
• clears heat in liver and blood
Sang Bai Pi: • relieves coughing and clears heat in the lungs
Sang Zhi: • expels wind and activates the channels
Sang Shen: • replenishes yin and nourishes blood

TYPICAL CHINESE DOSE
⅙₀–½ ounce (5–15 grams)

COMBINATIONS
Sang Zhi is used with Wei Ling Xian (Chinese clematis) for rheumatic pains linked to wind-damp; Sang Ye with Ju Hua (chrysanthemum), Bo He (field mint), Jie Geng (balloon flower), and Lian Qiao (forsythia) for external windheat. Sang Shen with He Shou Wu (flowery knotweed) for deficient liver and kidneys.

MULBERRY

Cautions

Sang Bai Pi and Sang Ye should not be used in cold conditions, and Sang Shen should be avoided in cases of diarrhea.

Bì Syndrome and Arthritis

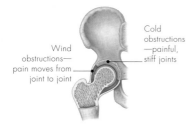

Wind obstructions—pain moves from joint to joint

Cold obstructions—painful, stiff joints

Joints

TCM treats the causes of arthritic disorders as wind, cold, hot, or damp obstructions, rather than wear and tear.

TCM suggests four prime causes for arthritic pains. In each case the specific Bì syndrome (Bì Zheng) has different external pathogens affecting the limb meridians to cause obstructions:

• wind obstructions; the shifting nature of wind is the key differentiator and pain moves from joint to joint;

• cold obstructions; fixed, stiff joints with severe pain that is worse in cold weather and during movement;

• damp obstructions, where the pain is usually fixed and there is swelling and numbness in the affected joints;

• hot obstructions, characterized by joint swelling, pain, and feverishness. These forms of Bì Zheng usually exist in combination within the osteoarthritis or rheumatic pains of old age—a combination of wind-cold-damp. Rheumatoid arthritis is usually a hot form, sometimes in heat-damp or wind-heat combinations.

Fu Zi Tang

A typical formula for arthritis associated with cold-damp combines warming, drying remedies with liver and Qi tonics. The liver is linked to the tendons so it may be weak or deficient too.

Fu Zi (prepared aconite) ¼ ounce (6 grams);

Bai Zhu (white atractylodes) ⅓ ounce (9 grams);

Ren Shen (Korean ginseng) ¹⁄₁₀ ounce (3 grams);

Bai Shao Yao (white peony) ¼ ounce (6 grams);

Fu Ling (tuckahoe) ⅓ ounce (9 grams).

Fu Zi (aconite) is a toxic herb that is used in TCM for extreme cold conditions. Because the root is so poisonous it must be prepared first. This is done by decocting with ginger or by mixing with salt, brown sugar, or sulfur in a lengthy and traditional process. It is not an herb for use by the untrained.

Gui Zhi Shao Yao Zhi Mu Tang

This is for wind-cold-damp Bi syndrome and uses warm, drying herbs modified with Zhi Mu (a cold, bitter remedy). Again, liver and kidney tonics are included:

Gui Zhi (cinnamon twigs) 1/4 ounce (6 grams);

Bai Shao Yao (white peony) ¼ ounce (6 grams);

Zhi Mu (*Anemarrhena asphelaidaa*) ¼ ounce (6 grams);

Ma Huang (ephedra) ¼ ounce (6 grams);

Bai Zhu (white atractylodes) ¼ ounce (6 grams);

Fu Zi (prepared aconite) ¼ ounce (6 grams);

Gan Cao (licorice root) ½10 ounce (3 grams);

Sheng Jiang (fresh ginger) 3 pieces.

This remedy is used when symptoms include pain in the joints with swelling in a shifting pattern in affected areas. This is not a recipe suitable for home use.

CANG ER ZI Cocklebur

Cang Er Zi literally means "deep green ear seeds" and it is one of the herbs used to clear wind-damp. Wind-damp often leads to nasal congestion and studies in China have shown that the herb is a very effective antimucosal, even for long-standing cases of allergic rhinitis. It was first listed in the "Thousand Ducat Prescriptions" (*Qian Jin Yao Fang*) written by Sun Simiao around 620AD.

At A Glance

BOTANICAL NAME
Xanthium strumarium

COMMON NAME
Cocklebur

FAMILY
Compositae

PART USED
Fruit

TASTE
Pungent, bitter

CHARACTER
Warm, toxic

MERIDIANS
Lung

ACTIONS
Antibacterial, anticatarrhal, antifungal, antirheumatic, antispasmodic, analgesic

TRADITIONAL USES
• to open the nasal passages
• to dispel wind-damp—including Bì syndrome (arthritis/rheumatism) and skin irritations
• to relieve pain due to exterior wind

TYPICAL CHINESE DOSE
⅒–⅓ ounce (3–9 grams)

COMBINATIONS
Cang Er Zi (cocklebur) is used with Bo He (field mint) and Jin Yin Hua (honeysuckle) for sinus problems in chronic wind-heat syndromes; with Huang Qin (baical skullcap) for acute wind-heat patterns; and with Jin Ying Zi (Cherokee rose) and Wu Wei Zi (schisandra) for allergic rhinitis.

COCKLEBUR

Cautions

Not to be used for headache or arthritic pains associated with anemia or blood deficiency. It contains a chemical called xanthostrumarin, which may be toxic in high doses, leading to convulsions.

WU JIA PI

Siberian ginseng This herb came to fame in the West in the 1950s when it was extensively used by Soviet athletes to increase stamina and enhance performance. It has been used in China for at least 2,000 years and was recommended by Shen Nong for abdominal pains, Qi weakness, and sores, while he claimed it also enabled the "lame child to walk instantly."

At A Glance

BOTANICAL NAME
Eleutherococcus senticosus

COMMON NAME
Siberian ginseng

FAMILY
Araliaceae

PART USED
Root bark

TASTE
Pungent

CHARACTER
Warm

MERIDIANS
Liver, kidney

ACTIONS
Tonic, stimulant, combats stress, antiviral, lowers blood sugar, immunostimulant

TRADITIONAL USES
• expels wind-dampness and strengthens sinews and bones
• transforms dampness and reduces swelling

TYPICAL CHINESE DOSE
⅓–½ ounce (9–15 grams)

COMBINATIONS
Used with Chen Pi (tangerine peel), Fu Ling (tuckahoe), and ginger peel in Wu Pi San as a diuretic remedy; and with Wei Ling Xian (Chinese clematis) and Qin Jiao (large-leaved gentian) for muscle pains and spasms associated with wind-damp. Although the Chinese only use the root bark, the whole root is used in the West as a tonic remedy to combat stress.

SIBERIAN GINSENG

Cautions

Avoid in deficient yin (see pages 68–69) with heat signs.

Hot Bì Syndromes

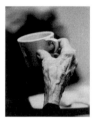

Arthritic hands
*Rheumatoid arthritis may
be regarded as hot bì syndrome
in TCM. It commonly affects
the joints of the hands.*

Arthritic problems associated with hot inflamed joints, feverishness, or associated skin rashes would be attributed in TCM to a hot obstruction in the meridians. Rheumatoid arthritis is a severe systemic disease that leads to joint deformity in the long term and this is in the hot category. The sort of arthritis that is linked to psoriasis (a chronic skin disorder), and which the West often attributes to autoimmune problems (where the body starts to destroy its own cells), would also be described as a hot condition.

Wind-heat Bì syndrome is characterized by sore joints, stiffness, and a difficulty in moving, often accompanied by a fever and thirst. Damp-heat Bì syndrome also has fever and thirst, but skin eruptions are more likely and the joints will be more swollen and painful. In rheumatoid arthritis there is often a changing pattern of symptoms and either of these varieties could be more dominant.

Er Miao San

This is the basic formula for treating damp-heat forms of Bì syndrome, especially those affecting the lower back with knee pains linked to weakened liver energies. It is made up of:

Huang Bai (amur cork tree) ¼ ounce (6 grams);

Cang Zhu (gray atractylodes) ⅓ ounce (9 grams).

Huai Niu Xi (two-toothed amaranthus) can also be added as additional support for the liver and knees and the mix is then known as San Miao San. If dampness is a major problem, then Yi Yi Ren (Job's tears) is added to the mix.

Bai Hu Jia Gui Zhi Tang

This decoction is used for treating arthritic pains associated with wind, heat, and dampness where the symptoms include painful, swollen joints. It is made up of:

Gui Zhi (cinnamon twigs) ¼ ounce (6 grams);

Shi Gao (gypsum or calcium sulfate) ⁷⁄₁₀ ounce (20 grams);

Zhi Mu (*Anemarrhena aspheloides*) ⅓ ounce (9 grams);

Jing Mi (rice seed) ½ ounce (15 grams);

Gan Cao (licorice root) ¹⁄₁₀ ounce (3 grams).

Shi Gao is one of the main minerals used in TCM. It is very cold and is used to clear heat in interior syndromes such as stomach fire problems, asthmatic conditions, and heat obstructing the meridians.

Rice is, of course, China's staple food. Jing Mi (rice seed), Gu Ya (sprouted rice), and Nuo Dao Gen Xu (rhizomes) are all used in TCM. Jing Mi is an energy tonic for the spleen and stomach, Gu Ya is mainly for food stagnation, while Nuo Dao Gen Xu is for feverish conditions linked to kidney weakness.

QIN JIAO Large-leaved gentian

Shen Nong described this variety of gentian as "bitter and balanced." It was considered useful for treating various cold, heat, and damp conditions adding that it "precipitates water and disinhibits urination," though there is no evidence that it is a diuretic. Several other species of gentian are used in Chinese herbalism including Long Dan Cao (Japanese gentian), which is largely used for liver problems.

At A Glance

BOTANICAL NAME
Gentiana macrophylla

COMMON NAME
Large-leaved gentian

FAMILY
Gentianaceae

PART USED
Root

TASTE
Pungent, bitter

CHARACTER
Neutral

MERIDIANS
Stomach, liver, gallbladder

ACTIONS
Antibacterial, anti-inflammatory, analgesic, sedative, increases blood sugar, lowers blood pressure

TRADITIONAL USES
• to eliminate wind-dampness
• to clear heat and damp in deficient yin

TYPICAL CHINESE DOSE
1/10–1/3 ounce (3–9 grams)

COMBINATIONS
Used with Huang Qin (baical skullcap) and Cang Zhu (gray atractylodes) for damp-heat and jaundice; with Dang Gui (Chinese angelica) and Bai Shao Yao (white peony) for deficient blood syndromes; and with Huo Ma Ren (cannabis seeds) for constipation that is associated with dry intestines.

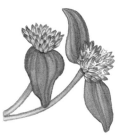

LARGE-LEAVED GENTIAN

Cautions

Avoid in polyuria (frequent urination), diarrhea, or general debility.

WEI LING XIAN Chinese

clematis European varieties of clematis may be used in homeopathy although rarely in herbal medicine. The Chinese variety has been used in TCM for 1,000 years, and was first mentioned in "Medicinal Recipes" (*Yao Pu*) by Hou Ning Ji. The herb has the valuable first-aid use of softening fish bones and is taken with vinegar and brown sugar as a household remedy if someone has fish bones lodged in the throat.

At A Glance

BOTANICAL NAME
Clematis chinensis

COMMON NAME
Chinese clematis

FAMILY
Ranunculaceae

PART USED
Root

TASTE
Pungent, salty

CHARACTER
Warm

MERIDIANS
Urinary bladder

ACTIONS
Antibacterial, antitumor, lowers blood sugar levels, analgesic, limits flow of urine

TRADITIONAL USES
• to dispel wind and dampness
• to invigorate the circulation of Qi in all the meridians

TYPICAL CHINESE DOSE
⅒–⅖ ounce (3–12 grams)

COMBINATIONS
Used with Huai Niu Xi (two-toothed amaranthus) or Du Huo (pubescent angelica) for joint pains in the lower half of the body due to wind-damp; and with herbs focused on the upper part of the body (e.g. Qiang Huo, *Notopterygium incisium*) for rheumatic pains in the upper back and shoulders.

CHINESE CLEMATIS

Cautions

Avoid in deficient blood syndromes.

SECRETS OF CHINESE HERBAL MEDICINE

Herbs to Clear Phlegm and Dampness

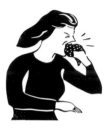

Phlegm

Phlegm problems in TCM include many more disorders than our Western concept of phlegm as the sputum produced when we cough.

Dampness in TCM can be both the external damp "evil" contributing to various arthritic problems as well as the internal collection of fluids in the body.

External damp can enter the interior and cause a variety of syndromes. Combined with heat it can lead to painful urinary problems (Lin Bing), damp feverish conditions (Shi Wen), or irritant skin rashes associated with damp-heat (Chuang Zhen). Treatment is usually

with a combination of herbs that dry the dampness and others that clear the heat.

The Chinese believe there are two sorts of phlegm—visible and invisible. The visible is familiar as sputum, but the invisible type collects inside the body and can be both a product and cause of disease. Spleen Qi deficiency will lead to the production of phlegm that will then move toward the heart causing a blockage. This can be a cause of both heart disorders and psychological problems, such as schizophrenia, since the heart is the key focus for mental activity.

Treating phlegm and dampness

Draining dampness involves increasing production of urine, so the herbs would be described in the West as diuretics. This group includes Fu Ling (tuckahoe), Yi Yi Ren (Job's tears), Mu Tong (chocolate vine), Bei Xia (yam), Yu Mi Shu (maize), and Ze Xie (water plantain). Cold or damp phlegm is treated with warming herbs. Cold phlegm often affects the stomach and manifests as vomiting and nausea so many of these remedies are also used for digestive problems. The group includes Ban Xia (pinellia), Xuan Fu Hua (Japanese elecampane), Jie Geng (balloon flower), Xing Ren (apricot seeds), Kuan Dong Hua (coltsfoot flowers), Zi Su Zi (perilla seeds), and Sang Bai Pi (mulberry root bark).

Hot or dry phlegm needs to be treated with cool herbs. This sort affects the lungs so the herbs are often antitussive or expectorant to relieve coughs. The group includes Chuan Bei Mu (tendrilled fritillary), Zhe Bei Mu (fritillary), several bamboo extracts, and parts of the snake gourd.

More Information

For more information see: **Ban Xia**, page 179; **Chuan Bei Mu**, page 194; **Fu Ling**, page 174; **Jie Geng**, page 191; **Sang Bai Pi**, page 163; **Xuan Fu Hua**, page 198; **Yi Yi Ren**, page 175; **Ze Xie**, page 178; **Zhe Bei Mu**, page 195; **lung**, pages 192–193; **spleen**, pages 176–177; **phlegm**, pages 172–173.

FU LING

Tuckahoe Fu Ling is one of the many fungi that are used in Chinese medicine and it is particularly effective as a diuretic. As well as the main body of the fungus, the brown skin (Fu Ling Pi) is used solely as a diuretic and the central part of the sclerotium is sometimes separated out as Fu Shen and used as a stronger sedative and calming remedy for the heart.

At A Glance

BOTANICAL NAME
Wolfiporia cocos

COMMON NAME
Tuckahoe, Indian bread, China root

FAMILY
Polyporaceae

PART USED
Sclerotium of the fungus that is usually found on the roots of pine trees

TASTE
Sweet, neutral

CHARACTER
Neutral

MERIDIANS
Lung, spleen, heart, urinary bladder

ACTIONS
Stimulates urine flow, sedative, lowers blood sugar levels

TRADITIONAL USES
• to clear dampness and regulate water metabolism
• to strengthen the spleen, stomach, and middle Jiao; transforms phlegm
• to quiet the heart and calm Shen (spirit)

TYPICAL CHINESE DOSE
¼–³⁄₅ ounce (6–18 grams)

COMBINATIONS
Used with Ze Xie (water plantain), Bai Zhu (white atractylodes), and Gui Zhi (cinnamon twigs) for scanty urination, edema, or painful urinary dysfunction; with Ban Xia (pinellia), Chen Pi (tangerine peel), and Sheng Jiang (fresh ginger) for phlegm and fluid problems leading to abdominal bloating; and with Gan Cao (licorice root) for spleen and heart deficiency.

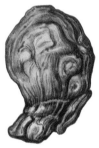

TUCKAHOE

Cautions

Avoid in cases of excessive urination or ptolapse of the urogenital organs.

YI YI REN Job's tears

Job's tears seeds (Yi Yi Ren) can be used in cooking in a similar way to pearl barley for making porridge and soups. The herb was listed by Shen Nong as a sweet tonic that helps the sinews "contract and stretch" and that combats wind-damp. He gave it the alternative name of Jie Le (woodworm eliminator) and recommended the root for intestinal worms.

At A Glance

BOTANICAL NAME
Coix lachryma-jobi

COMMON NAME
Job's tears

FAMILY
Graminae/Poaceae

PART USED
Seeds

TASTE
Sweet

CHARACTER
Cool

MERIDIANS
Spleen, stomach, lung, large intestine

ACTIONS
Muscle relaxant, antitumor, analgesic, sedative, lowers blood sugar, reduces fever

TRADITIONAL USES
• to resolve dampness and regulate water metabolism
• to tonify the spleen and stop diarrhea
• to clear inflammations and pus
• to expel wind-damp causing painful obstructions
• to clear damp-heat

TYPICAL CHINESE DOSE
⅓–1 ounce (9–30 grams)

COMBINATIONS
Used with Fu Ling (tuckahoe) and Bai Zhu (white atractylodes) in diarrhea linked to spleen deficiency; with Ma Huang (ephedra), Xing Ren (apricot seeds), Shi Gao (gypsum), and Gan Cao (licorice root) in Ma Xing Shi Gan Tang for wind-damp problems and asthmatic conditions.

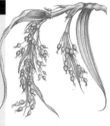

JOB'S TEARS

Cautions

Avoid during pregnancy.

Spleen and Stomach

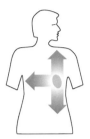

Food essence
The spleen circulates food essence, sending water to the kidneys and nutrients around the body.

The spleen (Pi) is one of the five Zang or solid organs. In TCM it is endowed with a number of functions that are very different from the Western view of the organ. It is basically seen as central to digestion and muscle development.

The spleen is traditionally believed to absorb the nutrients from food and then to stimulate the dispersal of this "food essence" through the body. If spleen Qi is strong the digestion and distribution of nutrients work well and the body is healthy. If it is weak then tissues become malnourished. The spleen performs the same function with water extracted from food, sending it through the body to reach the kidneys. This association with nutrition explains why the spleen is said to be responsible for building strong limbs and well-developed muscles. It is said to control the limbs and flesh, so muscular aches and pains or weakness can suggest spleen deficiency.

Strong spleen Qi is needed to keep blood flowing in the vessels. If it is weak then there may be hemorrhages or subcutaneous bleeding.

The spleen is involved in mental activities and is specifically responsible for "Yi." This is variously translated as intention, willpower, determination, or an awareness of the possibilities open to us to make changes in our lives.

The spleen's hollow partner

The stomach (Wei) is paired with the spleen; it takes in and digests food and is regarded in Chinese theory as the reservoir for food and water. Its effectiveness in starting the digestive process is seen as a function of stomach Qi. If it is strong then the "turbid" component from food is propelled to the small intestine. If it is weak, however, food tends to stagnate in the stomach.

The spleen and stomach are very closely associated—more so than the other Zang-Fu pairings—and the terms are sometimes used interchangeably. The stomach rules "descending" activities while the spleen controls "ascending" actions. The stomach sends nutrients and waste materials downward, while the spleen is involved in the upward transportation of water and has an aversion to dampness.

Functions of the Spleen

The spleen is said to:

- control digestion
- control the limbs and flesh
- keep blood in the blood vessels
- store intention or determination
- be linked to the mouth/appetite
- be reflected in the lips

ZE XIE

Water plantain Shen Nong included Ze Xie in his "superior class of herbs," declaring that this herb had the ability to "boost the Qi...and make one fat and strong" as well as to prolong life and "enable one to walk over water." Rather more moderate claims are made for the herb today—it is known to be an effective diuretic and liver remedy.

At A Glance

BOTANICAL NAME
Alisma plantago-aquatica

COMMON NAME
Water plantain

FAMILY
Alismataceae

PART USED
Tuber

TASTE
Sweet

CHARACTER
Cold

MERIDIANS
Kidney, urinary bladder

ACTIONS
Antibacterial, stimulates urine flow, lowers blood pressure, lowers blood sugar and cholesterol

TRADITIONAL USES
• to regulate water metabolism and resolve dampness
• to eliminate heat and dampness in the lower Jiao

TYPICAL CHINESE DOSE
⅒–⅖ ounce (3–12 grams)

COMBINATIONS
Ze Xie (water plantain) is used with Ban Xia (pinellia) for dampness in the middle Jiao associated with urinary problems and abdominal distension; and with Shu Di Huang (Chinese foxglove), Shan Zhu Yu (dogwood), Shan Yao (Chinese yam), Mu Dan Pi (tree peony), and Fu Ling (tuckahoe) in Liu Wei Di Huang Wan, which is used to strengthen liver and kidney yin.

WATER PLANTAIN

Cautions

Avoid in deficient kidney yang (see pages 68–69).

BAN XIA Pinellia

Ban Xia means "half summer," since the herb is traditionally collected during midsummer. It was listed in the *Shen Nong Ben Cao Jing* and is recommended for treating "cold damage" and, among other problems, "rumbling intestines." It is a toxic plant and is usually soaked in tea or vinegar before use to neutralize its more potent constituents.

At A Glance

BOTANICAL NAME
Pinellia ternata

COMMON NAME
Pinellia

FAMILY
Araceae

PART USED
Tuber

TASTE
Pungent

CHARACTER
Warm

MERIDIANS
Lung, spleen, stomach

ACTIONS
Combats nausea and vomiting, relieves coughs, expectorant, lowers blood cholesterol levels; antidote for strychnine poisoning; one study suggests it may relieve toothaches

TRADITIONAL USES
• to clear phlegm and dampness
• to disperse lumps and swellings
• to reverse the flow of Qi

TYPICAL CHINESE DOSE
¼–⅓ ounce (6–9 grams)

COMBINATIONS
Fa Ban Xia is made by mixing Ban Xia with alum, licorice, and calcium carbonate as a phlegm remedy and Jiang Ban Xia is made by mixing it with alum and ginger for nausea and vomiting. Ban Xia is also combined with Chen Pi (tangerine peel) for vomiting and nausea due to stomach Qi imbalance, and with Huang Lian (Chinese gold thread) for abdominal distension due to hot and cold evils invading the stomach.

PINELLIA

Cautions

Avoid in pregnancy and blood disorders.

The San Jiao

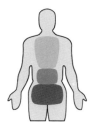

Triple burner

The San Jiao, or triple burner, can be divided into three sections, corresponding to the lower, middle, and upper sections of the torso.

The San Jiao—usually translated as the triple burner or three heater—is a Chinese concept dating back to the Yellow Emperor. It is an attempt to represent the body's digestive function.

The name literally means "three that burn" and this rather nebulous organ is sometimes listed as a sixth Fu or hollow yang organ along with the stomach, large intestine, small intestine, gallbladder, and urinary bladder of the five element model (see page 38). The San Jiao is paired with the pericardium (the sac around the heart) as a Zang organ. The San Jiao is described as a formless sewage system that transports and transforms nutrients while eliminating waste material; other early texts suggest that it supports various kinds of Qi.

The San Jiao can be a difficult concept for Westerners, since it combines not only the anatomic location of various organs, but also a view of digestive function that bears little resemblance to human physiology as it is now understood. The San Jiao is best regarded as a generalization of internal functions related to water regulation and digestion. It has three components:

• The upper Jiao, which relates to the chest above the diaphragm. It is associated with the heart and lungs.

• The middle Jiao, between the diaphragm and navel, which reflects the functions of the spleen and stomach.

• The lower Jiao, below the navel, is associated with the kidney and urinary bladder. The liver is also included here, reflecting the path of the liver meridian rather than the location of the organ.

Remedies for the San Jiao

Many herbs are indicated for strengthening the San Jiao and it can also be implicated in a variety of disorders. External wind-heat flooding the San Jiao can cause headaches and fever, while dampness in the middle burner (Zhong Jiao) is often linked to food stagnation and sluggish digestion.

Bu Zhong Yi Qi Tang

This remedy is used for weak spleen and stomach function and to strengthen yang (associated with the San Jiao).

Huang Qi (astragalus) ¼ ounce (6 grams);

Ren Shen (Korean ginseng) ¼ ounce (8 grams);

Bai Zhu (white atractylodes) ⅓ ounce (9 grams);

Gan Cao (licorice root) ¹⁄₁₀ ounce (3 grams);

Dang Gui (Chinese angelica) ¼ ounce (6 grams);

Sheng Ma (bugbane, cohosh) ¹⁄₁₀ ounce (3 grams);

Chai Hu (bupleurum) ¼ ounce (6 grams);

Chen Pi (tangerine peel) ¼ ounce (6 grams).

HUO XIANG

Patchouli Many Chinese medicinal herb names represent more than one species and Huo Xiang can also be *Agastache rugosa* (giant wrinkled hyssop). Whatever plant Huo Xiang happens to be, it is always classified as an aromatic to clear damp. The herb has been used since 500AD when it was listed in the *Ming Yi Bei Lu* (*Miscellaneous Records of Famous Physicians*).

At A Glance

BOTANICAL NAME
Pogostemon cablin

COMMON NAME
Patchouli

FAMILY
Labiatae/Lamiaceae

PARTS USED
Aerial parts

TASTE
Pungent

CHARACTER
Slightly warm

MERIDIANS
Lung, spleen, stomach

ACTIONS
Antibacterial, antifungal, induces sweating, digestive tonic

TRADITIONAL USES
• to transform dampness in the spleen and stomach
• to harmonize the middle Jiao and combat nausea
• to dispel cold

TYPICAL CHINESE DOSE
⅒–⅓ ounce (3–9 grams)

COMBINATIONS
Used with Huo Po (*Magnolia officinalis*), Chen Pi (tangerine peel), Bai Zhi (dahurian angelica), Zi Su Ye (perilla leaf), Fu Ling (tuckahoe), Bai Zhu (white atractylodes), Jie Geng (balloon flower), and other herbs in Huo Xiang Zheng Qi San for interior damp with wind-cold found in digestive upsets with diarrhea. Used with Huang Qin (baical skullcap), Lian Qiao (forsythia), Chuan Bei Mu (tendrilled fritillary), Bo He (field mint), and other herbs in Gan Lu Xiao Du Dan to clear interior damp and heat associated with fevers and acute gastroenteritis.

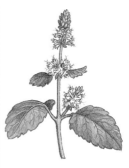

PATCHOULI

Cautions

Avoid in deficient yin (see pages 68–69) and stomach fire.

ROU DOU KOU Nutmeg

Nutmeg is familiar in the West as a kitchen seasoning, although it is a very potent herb that can cause delirium in high doses. Nutmeg has been used in TCM as a digestive remedy for the spleen and stomach since around 600AD when it was listed in the *Yao Xing Ben Cao* (*Materia Medica of Medicinal Properties*) by Zhen Quan.

At A Glance

BOTANICAL NAME
Myristica fragrans

COMMON NAME
Nutmeg

FAMILY
Myristaceae

PART USED
Seed (nut)

TASTE
Pungent

CHARACTER
Warm

MERIDIANS
Spleen, stomach, large intestine

ACTIONS
Antispasmodic, combats nausea and vomiting, appetite stimulant, anti-inflammatory, relieves gas and indigestion, digestive stimulant

TRADITIONAL USES
• to restrain leakage from the intestines and stop diarrhea
• to warm the spleen, stomach, and middle Jiao and regulate Qi flow

TYPICAL CHINESE DOSE
$\frac{1}{100}$–$\frac{1}{4}$ ounce (1–6 grams)

COMBINATIONS
Used with Bu Gu Zhi (scruf pea), Wu Zhu Yu (evodia), Wu Wei Zi (schisandra), Sheng Jiang (fresh ginger), and Da Zao (Chinese dates) in Si Shen Wan for "cock crow" diarrhea associated with kidney and spleen deficiency; and with Dang Shen (asiabell root), Bai Zhu (white atractylodes), and Gan Jiang (dried ginger) or with Ban Xia (pinellia) and Gan Jiang for cold deficient spleen and stomach appearing as chronic diarrhea with poor appetite.

NUTMEG

Cautions

Avoid in diarrhea caused by heat factors. Large single doses ($\frac{3}{10}$ ounce/7.5 grams) can produce dizziness, convulsions, or hallucinations. Avoid in pregnancy.

Food Stagnation

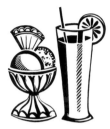

"Cold" foods

Food stagnation can be associated with a preference for "cold" foods such as fish, shellfish, ice creams, and cold drinks.

Food stagnation is a TCM syndrome that can be compared, in part, with our Western concept of indigestion, although it is more wide-ranging and complex. Food stagnation is associated with stagnant Qi caused by emotional imbalance as well as poor diet or eating habits. Rushed food and inadequate or excessive meals can all contribute to the problem.

Hot food stagnation is associated with bad breath, abdominal distension, and a preference for cold foods. It is usually caused by external evils moving inward to affect the spleen and stomach. It is generally treated with cooling herbs to clear the heat.

Cold food stagnation can be associated with a deficient spleen or stomach as well as attack by external cold caused by eating cold food. The Chinese will avoid eating ice cream or raw foods that are deemed too cold to risk. Cold food stagnation is characterized by nausea, excessive salivation or regurgitation of clear fluids, abdominal distension, and a preference for hot foods and drinks.

Herbs used for food stagnation include: Shan Zha (Chinese hawthorn); Mai Ya (barley sprouts); Gu Ya (rice sprouts); Shen Qu—medicated leaven, a very variable fermented mixture of wheat flour with the addition of various herbs and beans such as Cang Er Zi (cocklebur), Qing Hao (wormwood), Xing Ren (apricot seeds), adzuki beans, and water pepper; and Lai Fu Zi (radish seeds), which cause Qi to descend and transform phlegm.

Bao He Wan

These "pills for indigestion" are used to improve the stomach's digestive function and clear stagnant food; the basic remedy can be enhanced with additional cold, bitter herbs, usually Huang Qin (baical skullcap) and Huang Lian (Chinese gold thread), for hot food stagnation with bad breath. It contains:

Shan Zha (Chinese hawthorn) ⅓ ounce (9 grams);

Shen Qu (medicated leaven) ¼ ounce (6 grams);

Lai Fu Zi (radish seeds) ⅓ ounce (9 grams);

Ban Xia (pinellia) ¼ ounce (6 grams)

Chen Pi (tangerine peel) ⅒ ounce (3 grams);

Fu Ling (tuckahoe) ¼ ounce (6 grams);

Lian Qiao (forsythia) ¼ ounce (6 grams).

More Information

For more information see **Ban Xia**, page 179; **Cang Er Zi**, page 166; **Chen Pi**, page 82; **Da Huang**, page 154; **Fu Ling**, page 174; **Lian Qiao**, page 143; **Shan Zha**, page 186.

SHAN ZHA Chinese hawthorn

Hawthorn is mainly used in the West as a heart tonic and to normalize blood pressure. In contrast, the closely related Chinese species is seen as a digestive remedy, and therefore it is often used to treat food stagnation. It is also viewed as being a circulatory stimulant. It first appears in a fourteenth-century Chinese herbal entitled the *Ben Cao Yan Yi Bu Yi* written by Zhu Zhen Heng.

At A Glance

BOTANICAL NAME
Crataegus pinnatifida

COMMON NAME
Chinese hawthorn

FAMILY
Rosaceae

PART USED
Fruit

TASTE
Sour, sweet

CHARACTER
Slightly warm

MERIDIANS
Spleen, stomach, liver

ACTIONS
Antibacterial, lowers blood pressure, relaxes blood vessels, cardiac tonic, lowers cholesterol levels

TRADITIONAL USES
• to eliminate food stagnation and improve digestion
• to invigorate blood circulation and clear blood stagnation

TYPICAL CHINESE DOSE:
⅓–½ ounce (9–15 grams)

COMBINATIONS:
Used with Rou Dou Gou (nutmeg) and Bian Dou (hyacinth beans) for abdominal distension and pain with diarrhea linked to food stagnation; with Dan Shen (Chinese sage) for chest pains linked to blood stagnation in the heart channel; and with Chuan Xiong (Sichuan lovage) and Dang Shen (asiabell root) for stagnant blood causing menstrual or postpartum pain.

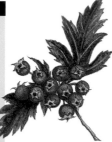

CHINESE HAWTHORN

Cautions

Use cautiously in cases of deficient spleen and stomach and if there is acid regurgitation.

CANG ZHU — Gray atractylodes

Cang Zhu is one of the main herbs for clearing dampness—both for internal damp problems associated with the spleen and for external damp. It was first listed in the *Zhong Lei Ben Cao* (*Materia Medica Arranged According to Pattern*) written by Tang Shen Wei around 1082. The famous sixteenth-century herbalist Li Shi Zhen recommended fumigation with Cang Zhu during epidemics as an important preventative.

At A Glance

BOTANICAL NAME
Atractylodes chinensis

COMMON NAME
Gray atractylodes

FAMILY
Compositae

PART USED
Rhizome

TASTE
Pungent, bitter

CHARACTER
Warm

MERIDIANS
Spleen, stomach

ACTIONS
Relieves gas and indigestion; induces sweating; increases excretion of sodium and potassium salts although it does not stimulate urine flow

TRADITIONAL USES
• to dry dampness and tonify the spleen
• to expel external wind, damp, and cold
• to clear dampness in the San Jiao

TYPICAL CHINESE DOSE
1/18–1/8 ounce (3–9 grams)

COMBINATIONS
Used with Hou Po (*Magnolia officinalis*) and Chen Pi (tangerine peel) in Ping Wei San for dampness in the spleen causing severe indigestion with diarrhea. Also with Ze Xie (water plantain), Fu Ling (tuckahoe), Gui Zhi (cinnamon twigs), Hou Po, Chen Pi (tangerine peel), and other herbs in Wei Ling Tang to regulate spleen and stomach Qi and clear dampness.

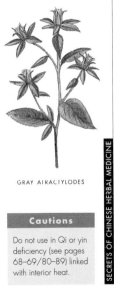

GRAY ATRACTYLODES

Cautions

Do not use in Qi or yin deficiency (see pages 68–69/80–89) linked with interior heat.

Dampness and Phlegm Syndromes

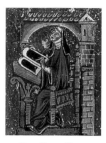

Gao Liang Jiang
The eleventh-century German mystic, Hildegard of Bingen, used Chinese herbs to treat angina.

Excess dampness leading to fluid collecting in the body is seen in TCM as a cause of edema and fluid congestion. Normal metabolism of body fluids (Jin-Ye) can become obstructed and congested and this can be a factor in various respiratory and digestive problems linked to dampness.

Phlegm can be regarded as a more complex variety of dampness and is the accumulation of thick fluid in the respiratory or digestive systems. Phlegm production is associated with the spleen's role in separating the clear and turbid fluids produced during digestion. Phlegm tends to be stored by the lungs, hence its manifestation in productive coughing. Asthma is also associated with excess phlegm and its characteristic wheeze is described as the "sound of phlegm."

Typical symptoms of phlegm syndrome include a thick and greasy coating to the tongue and a slippery or wiry pulse. Other symptoms will depend on where the phlegm is concentrated. If it is in the stomach it will lead to nausea and vomiting. If it is in the lung there will be coughing and shortness of breath. In the heart, there will be heart problems or mental disturbances, and so on.

Phlegm in the heart channel

The Chinese suggest that heart attacks and angina pectoris are caused by phlegm in the heart channel. Treatment aims to clear the phlegm with aromatic herbs while regulating spleen function to resolve the phlegm. It would include Ban Xia (pinellia); Chen Pi (tangerine peel), Zhi Ke (ripe bitter orange), Hou Po (bark of *Magnolia officinalis*), Fu Ling (tuckahoe), and Bai Zhu (white atractylodes), which are mainly digestive remedies aimed at normalizing spleen function and clearing dampness.

Chinese practitioners also prescribe pills containing Yan Hu Suo (bulbus corydalis), Gao Liang Jiang (galangal), Bi Ba (long pepper), Tan Xiang (sandalwood), and other herbs for angina pains. Gao Liang Jiang was used in eleventh-century Germany by Hildegard of Bingen for the same problem.

More Information

For more information see **body fluids (Jin-Ye)**, pages 100–101; **heart**, pages 108–109; **lung**, pages 192–193; **spleen**, pages 176–177; **stomach**, pages 176–177; **Ban Xia**, page 179; **Bai Zhu**, page 94; **Chen Pi**, page 82; **Fu Ling**, page 174; **Yan Hu Suo**, page 107.

BAI GUO

Ginkgo The leaves of the ginkgo tree have become very popular in the West over the past decade as a circulatory stimulant recommended for all kinds of conditions from varicose veins to the hardening of the arteries. In China only the seeds are used. They are available under a variety of names—Bai Guo, Yin Xing, or Yin Guo—all usually translated as "white seeds." The plant was first listed in 1350 in the *Household Materia Medica*, which was written by Wu Rui.

At A Glance

BOTANICAL NAME
Ginkgo biloba

COMMON NAME
Ginkgo, maidenhair tree

FAMILY
Ginkgoaceae

PARTS USED
Seeds

TASTE
Sweet, bitter, astringent

CHARACTER
Neutral

MERIDIANS
Lung, kidney

ACTIONS
Astringent, antifungal, antibacterial

TRADITIONAL USES:
• to consolidate lung Qi and relieve asthma
• to stop discharges (astringent)
• to stabilize the lower Jiao

TYPICAL CHINESE DOSE
¼–⅓ ounce (6–9 grams)

COMBINATIONS
Used with Ma Huang (ephedra), Xuan Dong Hua (tussilago flower), Zi Su Zi (perilla seeds), Xing Ren (apricot seeds), Sang Bai Pi (mulberry root bark), Huang Qin (baical skullcap), Ban Xia (pinellia), and Gan Cao (licorice root) in Ding Chuan Tang (a decoction for asthma used for heat in the lung and asthmatic conditions). It is combined with Huang Bai (amur cork tree) and other herbs for vaginal discharges associated with damp-heat.

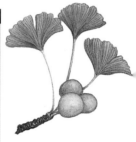

GINKGO

Cautions

Avoid in excess (Shi) syndromes. It is slightly toxic so avoid protracted use. Overdose can cause headaches and tremors—a combination of Gan Cao (licorice root) and ginkgo seed shells are used as an antidote.

JIE GENG Balloon flower

It is easy to see why balloon flowers are grown as a garden ornamental in the West. They have striking blue or white flowers that appear as a large balloon before fully opening out. The herb has been used as a cough remedy in Chinese medicine since the days of Shen Nong: he recommended it for "chest and rib pains as if stabbed by a knife" as well as "continual intestinal rumblings."

At A Glance

BOTANICAL NAME
Platycodon grandiflorum

COMMON NAME
Balloon flower

FAMILY
Campanulaceae

PART USED
Root

TASTE
Pungent, bitter

CHARACTER
Neutral

MERIDIANS
Lung

ACTIONS
Antifungal, antibacterial, expectorant, lowers blood sugar levels, reduces cholesterol levels

TRADITIONAL USES
• to circulate lung Qi
• to expel phlegm caused by wind-cold and wind-heat
• to direct other herbs upward
• to clear pus in lung or throat abscesses

TYPICAL CHINESE DOSE
1/10–1/3 ounce (3–9 grams)

COMBINATIONS
Used with Sang Ye (mulberry leaves), Ju Hua (chrysanthemum), Bo He (field mint), and Gan Cao (licorice root) in Sang Ju Yin, a remedy for coughs and colds; with Ban Xia (pinellia) for coughs linked to external wind-cold or chronic damp phlegm problems; with Bai Zhu (white atractylodes) for ulcerated abscesses; and with Gan Cao (licorice root) for sore throats and hoarseness caused by wind-heat.

BALLOON FLOWER

Cautions

Avoid in tuberculosis and if there is blood in the sputum.

Lung

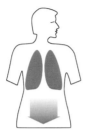

Water metabolism
The lungs are closely associated with water metabolism in TCM.

Like the spleen, the lungs (Fei) are also classified with the solid Zang organs and are closely linked to body fluids and water metabolism.

TCM regards the lungs as responsible for respiration but they also have many other attributes. In Ayurvedic theory, breath is associated with vital energy, which can be strengthened by exercise and breathing. In Chinese tradition, QiGong is used in a similar way to strengthen energy levels through better breath control. Given this link, the Chinese belief that the "lungs control Qi" seems quite logical.

Qi is subdivided into many different categories and the lungs are particularly associated with "defense Qi" (Wei Qi), which they help to send to the body's surface to repel invading evils.

The lung Qi tends to move downward so it encourages the flow of water and fluids (Jin-Ye) through the system to the kidney and urinary bladder. Lung problems are thus often blamed for edema and fluid retention in Chinese medicine.

Logically, the lungs are also connected with the nose—anatomically at the end of the respiratory tract—and also with the sense of smell. The connection with Wei Qi and surface energies highlights the view that the lungs are "seen in the skin and body hair." Healthy, glowing skin indicates strong lung Qi.

As with the other Zang organs, the lungs also have a spiritual aspect. In this case it is *Po*, sometimes translated as "vitality," which is associated more with the physical side of concentration rather than thought processes.

Large intestine

The large intestine (Da Chang) is associated with the lungs and, like the other fu (hollow) organs, is mainly involved with transportation and transformation. It is involved in compacting the solid wastes from our food, so the Chinese describe it as "governing body fluid."

If the large intestine fails to reabsorb sufficient moisture, stools become watery, causing diarrhea. Blockages in the large intestine—as in constipation —are believed to interfere with the descending function of lung Qi.

Functions of the Lungs

The lungs are said to:

- control Qi

- be responsible for respiration

- maintain the downward flow of fluid, regulate water circulation

- store vitality or "animal energy"

- be linked to the nose

- be seen in the skin and hair

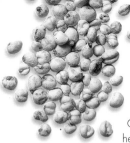

CHUAN BEI MU Tendrilled

fritillary Chuan Bei Mu is a comparative newcomer to TCM. It was introduced around 1750 during the Qing dynasty (1644–1911) and originally listed in an herbal from South Yunnan province. The plant is similar in action to Zhi Bei Mu (see opposite) but is more nourishing and moistening for the lung. It is commonly used in chronic respiratory problems, such as tuberculosis, and for less productive coughs. Chuan in Chinese plant names usually indicates that the herb comes from the Sichuan province. This particular herb's name translates as "shell mother of Sichuan."

At A Glance

BOTANICAL NAME
Fritillaria cirrhosa

COMMON NAME
Tendrilled fritillary

FAMILY
Liliaceae/Aloaceae

PART USED
Bulb

TASTE
Bitter, sweet

CHARACTER
Slightly cold

MERIDIANS
Lung, heart

ACTIONS
Relieves coughs, lowers blood pressure, muscle relaxant

TRADITIONAL USES
• to resolve phlegm and relieve cough
• to nourish and moisten the lung
• to disperse lumps and hard swellings

TYPICAL CHINESE DOSE
1/10–1/3 ounce (3–9 grams)

COMBINATIONS
Chuan Bei Mu is used with Fu Ling (tuckahoe) and other herbs for painful obstructions associated with blockages in the channels; with Zhe Bei Mu (fritillary) for abscesses; and with Xing Ren (apricot seeds) for coughing and wheezing with copious sputum.

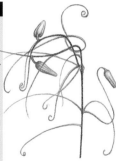

TENDRILLED FRITILLARY

Cautions

Avoid in deficient spleen or stomach syndromes.

ZHE BEI MU Fritillary

Zhe Bei Mu is one of the more important herbs used to clear the hot phlegm that is responsible for acute lung problems and productive coughs with thick yellow sputum. It is stronger in action than Chuan Bei Mu (tendrilled fritillary) and is more suitable for acute conditions such as asthma and bronchitis. Traditionally it was also used to disperse hard swellings and it has been used in breast-cancer treatments.

At A Glance

BOTANICAL NAME
Fritillaria verticillata

COMMON NAME
Fritillary

FAMILY
Liliaceae/Aloaceae

PART USED
Bulb

TASTE
Bitter

CHARACTER
Cold

MERIDIANS
Lung, heart

ACTIONS
Relieves coughs, lowers blood pressure, muscle relaxant

TRADITIONAL USES
• to clear and transform heat and phlegm
• to resolve coughs
• to disperse hard lumps and swellings

TYPICAL CHINESE DOSE
⅒–⅓ ounce (3–9 grams)

COMBINATIONS
Used with Lian Qiao (forsythia) and Niu Bang Zi (burdock) for acute coughs associated with external wind-heat; with Xuan Shen (ningpo figwort) and Xia Ku Cao (self-heal) for abscesses and swellings associated with phlegm fire; with Jin Yin Hua (honeysuckle), Pu Gong Ying (Chinese dandelion), and with Ju Hua (chrysanthemum) for abscesses and swellings due to fire poisons.

FRITILLARY

Cautions

Avoid in deficient spleen patterns.

Treating Lung Disorders

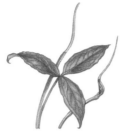

Pinellia

Ban Xia, pinellia, is a warm remedy to help clear interior cold and ease a stuffy nose and chest.

The lungs are so closely associated with the body's exterior surface and the nose that it is hardly surprising that they are a target for invasion by external wind-cold and wind-heat evils.

Invasion by wind-cold

Wind-cold that moves inside progresses from the sort of common cold that the attacking evil would cause, and increases the watery nasal mucus and causes a cough with white mucuslike sputum. In the West this might be labeled as a chest infection or simply a bad cold. A typical prescription would be Xing Su San which includes:

Xing Ren (apricot seeds) ¼ ounce (6 grams);

Zi Su Ye (perilla leaf) ¼ ounce (6 grams);

Zhi Ke (ripe bitter orange) ¼ ounce (6 grams);

Jie Geng (balloon flower) ¼ ounce (6 grams);

Qian Hu (*Peucedanum praeruptorum*) ¼ ounce (6 grams);

Chen Pi (tangerine peel) ⅒ ounce (3 grams);

Ban Xia (pinellia) ¼ ounce (6 grams);

Fu Ling (tuckahoe) ⅓ ounce (9 grams);

Sheng Jiang (fresh ginger) ⅒ ounce (3 grams);

Gan Cao (licorice root) ⅒ ounce (3 grams);

Da Zao (Chinese dates) 3 pieces.

This is a warming, diaphoretic (induces sweating) mixture.

Excessive sadness

The emotions associated with the lungs are grief and sadness and these may also be the cause of coughlike symptoms. Excess of these emotions can weaken the lungs and lead to Qi deficiency. This can be a cause of bronchitis or asthmatic conditions and it is not that unusual for a bereavement to trigger this sort of syndrome. Typical symptoms include shortness of breath, cough or wheeziness, copious thin sputum, tiredness, a weak-sounding voice, a pale or dry tongue with white coating, and an empty and weak pulse. One of the most effective herbs for this sort of lung Qi deficiency is Ren Shen (Korean ginseng). It can be used singly or within Sheng Mai San (activate vascular system powder). This contains:

Ren Shen ¼ ounce (6 grams);

Mai Men Dong (lilyturf) ¼ ounce (6 grams);

Wu Wei Zi (schisandra) ¼ ounce (6 grams).

More Information

For more information see **Ban Xia**, page 179; **Chen Pi**, page 82; **Da Zao**, page 95; **Fu Ling**, page 174; **Gan Cao**, page 90; **Jie Geng**, page 191; **Ren Shen**, page 86; **Sheng Jiang**, page 146; **wind-heat**, pages 56–57; lung, pages 192–193; phlegm, pages 172–173, **seven emotions**, pages 132–133.

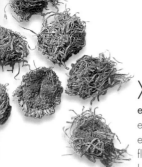

XUAN FU HUA Japanese elecampane

While the root of European elecampane (*Inula helenium*) is preferred as an effective expectorant and tonic, the Chinese use the flowers of this related species in a similar way. The herb is included among Shen Nong's "medium class" remedies and he recommended it for damp and cold problems. He also gave it an alternative name of Sheng Zhan, which means "profound clearness."

At A Glance

BOTANICAL NAME
Inula brittanica

COMMON NAME
Japanese elecampane, yellow starwort

FAMILY
Compositae/Asteraceae

PART USED
Flowerheads

TASTE
Salty

CHARACTER
Warm

MERIDIANS
Lung, spleen, stomach, large intestine

ACTIONS
Antibacterial, nervous stimulant, digestive stimulant

TRADITIONAL USES
• to redirect upwardly flowing lung and stomach Qi
• to resolve stagnation of phlegm in the lung

TYPICAL CHINESE DOSE
1/10–1/3 ounce (3–9 grams)

COMBINATIONS
It is combined with Ren Shen (Korean ginseng), Ban Xia (pinellia), Sheng Jiang (fresh ginger), Da Zao (Chinese dates), and Dai Zhe Shi (the mineral hematite) in Xuan Fu Dai Zhe Tang for stomach Qi problems.

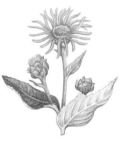

JAPANESE ELECAMPANE

Cautions

Avoid excessive use in deficiency syndromes.

XING REN Bitter apricot

Apricot seeds have been used as a medicinal herb since the sixth century and were first mentioned in the *Ben Cao Jing Ji Zhu* by Tao Hong-Jing around 500AD. They are used to relieve coughs and wheezing, and modern research has confirmed their efficacy as antitussive and anti-asthmatic. However, apricot seeds contain amygdalin, which breaks down in the body to form hydrocyanic acid which, in high doses, can be toxic.

At A Glance

BOTANICAL NAME
Prunus armeniaca

COMMON NAME
Bitter apricot

FAMILY
Rosaceae

PART USED
Seeds

TASTE
Bitter

CHARACTER
Slightly warm, slightly toxic

MERIDIANS
Lung, large intestine

ACTIONS
Relieves coughs, anti-asthmatic, antibacterial, antiparasitic, analgesic

TRADITIONAL USES
• to relieve coughs and stop wheezing
• to lubricate the intestines

TYPICAL CHINESE DOSE
1/10–1/3 ounce (3–9 grams)

COMBINATIONS
Xing Ren is used with Zi Su Ye (perilla leaf) for dry coughs associated with wind-cold; with Sang Ye (mulberry leaves) for non-productive coughs caused by wind-heat; with Ma Huang (ephedra) for conditions with wheezing; and with Huo Ma Ren (cannabis seeds) as a laxative for deficient, dry intestines.

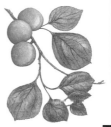

BITTER APRICOT

Cautions

Avoid in cases of coughs caused by deficient yin. Overdose can be fatal: deaths have been reported in adults eating 60 seeds and in children eating only 10.

Herbs for Essence

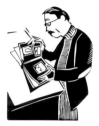

Jing

*Jing diminishes with age and
its lack is blamed in TCM for poor
hearing and eyesight, memory
loss, and graying hair.*

Jing, or vital essence, is one of the five "fundamental substances" of Chinese medicine, playing an important role in our creativity and reproduction. Jing is linked to the kidneys, where it is stored. Many of the factors associated with the kidney, such as head hair and hearing, also reflect the state of Jing.

Our congenital Jing is fixed at birth and erodes during our lifetimes. Signs of aging, such as hearing problems and graying hair, are thus seen as aspects of this run down in Jing. Jing is also essential for reproduction and its decay

is characterized, in women, by the onset of menopause, which is often treated in TCM as kidney weakness. Jing is also believed to produce bone marrow, which Chinese medicine associates with the brain (described as the "sea of the marrow"). This explains why Jing is associated with creativity. Poor memory, lack of concentration, or any sort of brain damage might be blamed on a weakness in bone marrow due to Jing deficiency and be treated with kidney tonics. The same applies to reproductive problems like impotence or miscarriage.

Herbs to strengthen Jing

Jing contains both yin and yang. When compared with active, external Qi, it is yin in character; when contrasted to internal, passive Xue (blood), it is yang.

When Jing is deficient, both the yin and yang of the body can be diminished. The first indication of Jing weakness is kidney deficiency—premature aging, poor teeth, poor memory, sexual dysfunction, and so on. As symptoms progress the Jing deficiency may appear to be more yin or yang in character—impotence in yang deficiency or vaginal dryness if yin dominates, for example.

Herbs to strengthen Jing are generally kidney tonics and many are associated with longevity and countering signs of aging. Both Nu Zhen Zi (glossy privet fruits) and He Shou Wu (flowery knotweed), for example, are traditionally said to darken prematurely graying hair.

Other useful Jing tonics include Hu Tao Ren (walnuts), Shi Hu (dendrobium orchid), Gou Qi Zi (wolfberry fruits), Shan Zhu Yu (dogwood), Wu Wei Zi (schisandra), Fu Pen Zi (Chinese raspberry), Jin Ying Zi (Cherokee rose), Shan Yao (Chinese yam), and Dong Chong Xia Cao (caterpillar fungus).

More Information

For more information see **Dong Chong Xia Cao**, page 62; **Fu Pen Zi**, page 207; **Gou Qi Zi**, page 118; **He Shou Wu**, page 114; **Hu Tao Ren**, page 67; **Jin Ying Zi**, page 206; **Nu Zhen Zi**, page 79; **Shi Hu**, page 75; **Shan Zhu Yu**, page 202; **Wu Wei Zi**, page 203.

SHAN ZHU YU Dogwood

Shan Zhu Yu is a type of dogwood sometimes grown as an ornamental in Western gardens. It was one of the herbs listed by Shen Nong over 2,000 years ago. He regarded it as being in the "middle class" declaring that it "warms the center and expels cold and damp." Today, it is used both as an astringent herb to stop bleeding and as a reproductive remedy to strengthen kidney energies. It is also a useful tonic for menopausal and menstrual problems.

At A Glance

BOTANICAL NAME
Cornus officinalis

COMMON NAME
Dogwood, Japanese cornelian cherry

FAMILY
Cornaceae

PART USED
Fruit

TASTE
Sour

CHARACTER
Warm

MERIDIANS
Liver, kidney

ACTIONS
Antibacterial, antifungal, stimulates urine flow, lowers blood pressure

TRADITIONAL USES
• to replenish the kidney and Jing
• to stabilize menstruation and replenish liver yin
• to stop bleeding and excessive sweating

TYPICAL CHINESE DOSE
¼–⅖ ounce (6–12 grams)

COMBINATIONS
In Liu Wei Di Huang Wan it is used with Shu Di Huang (Chinese foxglove), Shan Yao (Chinese yam), Ze Xie (water plantain), Mu Dan Pi (tree peony), and Fu Ling (tuckahoe) for menstrual, menopausal, and urinary tract problems. It is also used with warming remedies like Rou Gui (cinnamon bark) and Fu Zi (aconite) in Jin Gui Shen Qi Wan for menopausal, kidney, and respiratory problems such as asthma.

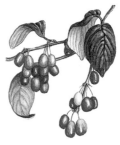

DOGWOOD

Cautions

Avoid in fire symptoms and deficient kidney yang; Shan Zhu Yu should not be combined with Jie Geng (balloon flower) or Fang Feng (ledebouriella).

WU WEI ZI Schisandra

Wu Wei Zi translates as "five taste seeds." It was once regarded as combining all five of the classic Chinese tastes, although the plant is characterized as "sour" in modern herbals. It is listed in the *Shen Nong Ben Cao Jing* as a Qi tonic and cough remedy that also "fortifies yin and boosts male's essence." It has long been regarded as an aphrodisiac and in folk tradition is taken as a cosmetic remedy to beautify the skin.

At A Glance

BOTANICAL NAME
Schisandra chinensis

COMMON NAME
Schisandra

FAMILY
Schisandraceae

PART USED
Fruit

TASTE
Sour

CHARACTER
Warm

MERIDIANS
Lung, heart, kidney

ACTIONS
Antibacterial, astringent, aphrodisiac, circulatory and digestive stimulant, sedative, expectorant, lowers blood pressure, tonic, uterine stimulant

TRADITIONAL USES
• to replenish Qi
• to promote body fluids
• to tonify kidney and heart and calm the spirit (Shen)
• to stop excessive sweating

TYPICAL CHINESE DOSE
⅓om–½ ounce (3–9 grams)

COMBINATIONS
Used with Gan Jiang (dried ginger), Ma Huang (ephedra), Gui Zhi (cinnamon twigs), and others for coughs and wheezing; with Ren Shen (Korean ginseng) and Mai Men Dong (lilyturf) in Sheng Mai San for lung weakness and chronic coughs; with Bai Zi Ren (tree of life seeds), Dan Shen (Chinese sage), Suan Zao Ren (wild date), and others in Tian Wang Bu Xin Dan to nourish heart and kidney yin in menopausal problems and insomnia.

SCHISANDRA

Cautions

Avoid in cases of internal heat and superficial syndromes.

The Kidney

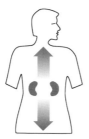

Water regulation

In TCM the kidneys are believed to send "clear fluid" to tissues, while "turbid" fluid is excreted as urine and sweat.

As you would expect, the kidneys (Shen) are associated with water metabolism and regulation in TCM. The Chinese, however, also link this function to the lungs. So, in turn, the kidneys are believed to play a part in coordinating the respiration process.

Chinese medicine also associates water regulation with "body fluids" (Jin-Ye). These are divided into "clear fluid," which circulates through the organs and tissues, and "turbid fluid," which is transformed into sweat and urine and is excreted. The kidneys send the clear fluid

upward and the turbid downward for disposal. They also help to direct the Qi flow downward, so aiding the work of the lung during inhalation. If kidney Qi is weak it can lead to breathing problems.

The kidney also transforms Jing into bone marrow, which spreads along the spinal cord to the brain—originally believed to be made of bone marrow. Through this connection the kidney is associated with head hair—an abundance of hair indicates healthy kidney Qi and strong Jing.

Teeth are seen as the bones' surplus, so are also ruled by the kidneys while the ears are the kidneys' external opening. The association with the reproductive system also links the kidneys to the outward genitalia. They also have a spiritual dimension, this time with Zhi, translated as "will" or "determination."

The kidneys during menopause

Menopausal problems are related to the natural run-down in the congenital Jing. Weakened kidneys fail to control fire so the heart becomes overexcited, leading to typical symptoms of night sweats, hot flashes, emotional upsets, palpitations, and tiredness. Erratic menstruation also affects blood and the liver. In most cases the main problem is an imbalance in kidney and liver energies, and herbal remedies focus on herbs to tonify Qi and Xue (blood). A typical prescription is Liu Wei Di Huang Wan:

Shu Di Huang (Chinese foxglove) ³⁄₅ ounce (18 grams);

Shan Zhu Yu (dogwood) ⅓ ounce (9 grams);

Shan Yao (Chinese yam) ⅓ ounce (9 grams);

Ze Xie (water plantain) ⅓ ounce (9 grams);

Mu Dan Pi (tree peony) ¼ ounce (6 grams);

Fu Ling (tuckahoe) ⅓ ounce (9 grams).

Functions of the Kidney

The kidney is said to:

- regulates water in the body
- coordinates respiration
- stores vital essence (Jing) and determination
- produces bone marrow
- Is seen in the hair and opens into the ear
- is linked to the ears and genitals

JIN YING ZI Cherokee rose

Roses are traditionally used in Western herbal medicine as astringents and to tonify "the skin and the soul." They have a similar standing in Chinese tradition as they are used to combat diarrhea and bleeding, and also to support Qi and Jing. Both Cherokee rosehip and Japanese rosebud (Mei Gui Hua—Japanese rose) are used in Chinese medicine. Mei Gui Hua is regarded as a Qi and blood tonic for the liver, while Jin Ying Zi is focused on the kidney.

At A Glance

BOTANICAL NAME
Rosa laevigata

COMMON NAME
Cherokee rose

FAMILY
Rosaceae

PART USED
Fruit (hips)

TASTE
Sweet, astringent

CHARACTER
Neutral

MERIDIANS
Kidney, urinary bladder, large intestine

ACTIONS
Astringent, antibacterial, antiviral, reduces cholesterol levels, tonifies uterus

TRADITIONAL USES
• to consolidate kidney Qi and retain Jing
• to restrain leakage from the intestines

TYPICAL CHINESE DOSE
1/10–1/3 ounce (3–9 grams)

COMBINATIONS
Used with herbs like Dang Shen (asiabell root), Shan Yao (Chinese yam), and Bai Zhu (white atractylodes) for diarrhea associated with deficient spleen; and with Mu Li (oyster shells) for impotence and reproductive problems associated with deficient kidney yin.

CHEROKEE ROSE

Cautions

Avoid in excess fire and heat syndromes.

FU PEN ZI Chinese raspberry

Raspberry leaves are mainly used in the West to ease childbirth and menstrual problems. The Chinese prefer the fruits but they are similarly used for the reproductive system, as a tonic for kidney yang in cases of impotence and premature ejaculation. Fu Pen Zi has been used in TCM for 1,500 years and first appeared in the *Ben Cao Jing Ji Zhu*, which was written by Tao Hong-Jing around 500AD.

At A Glance

BOTANICAL NAME
Rubus chingii

COMMON NAME
Chinese raspberry

FAMILY
Rosaceae

PART USED
Fruit

TASTE
Sweet, sour

CHARACTER
Slightly warm

MERIDIANS
Liver, kidney

ACTIONS
Estrogenic, astringent

TRADITIONAL USES
• to tonify liver and kidney
• to restrain Jing
• to brighten the eyes

TYPICAL CHINESE DOSE
⅓–½ ounce (9–15 grams)

COMBINATIONS
Used with Gou Qi Zi (wolfberry fruits), Wu Wei Zi (schisandra), and other herbs for impotence and spermatorrhea due to deficient kidneys; with Du Zhong (eucommia) for lower back pain linked to kidney weakness; and with black cardamom seeds (Yi Zhi Ren, *Alpinia oxyphylla*) and other herbs for urinary problems associated with lower Jiao deficiency.

CHINESE RASPBERRY

Cautions

Use cautiously in deficient yin syndromes (see pages 68–69); avoid if there is any difficulty urinating.

Herbs to Calm the Spirit

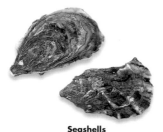

Seashells

Some types of seashells are used to calm the spirit, including oyster shells, which are crushed and made into pills.

Shen, or spirit, is one of the five fundamental substances of Chinese medicine. It is sometimes described as the "vitality behind Jing and Qi"—the substance that makes us human. Shen is considered to be yang in character. When grouped together with Jing and Qi they are known collectively as "the three treasures." Shen can seem a rather nebulous concept to Westerners since it combines mental awareness, vitality, and a certain inner calm.

Damage to Shen can be associated with mental illness and violent madness, as well as less dramatic problems such as muddled or slow thinking, insomnia, or forgetfulness. People who behave erratically or jump from one subject to another in conversation often suffer from some form of Shen disharmony.

Shen is stored in the heart and so problems associated with it can also manifest as physical heart signs, such as palpitations or a rapid heart beat.

Herbs to calm Shen

Herbs that in Western terms would be labeled as sedatives or tranquilizers are described in TCM as remedies to "settle and calm the spirit." Many are minerals or seashells and their heaviness is seen necessary to weigh upon the heart, calming and damping down the excesses of this fiery spirit.

Typical of the calming Shen remedies is Long Gu or dragon bones. This is derived from fossil bones—usually vertebra, finger, or toe bones—from long-dead mammals. Long Chi (fossilized teeth) are similarly valued. Rather less exotic is Mu Li (oyster shells), Ci Shi (magnetite, an ore containing iron oxide), Zhu Sha (cinnabar, mostly mercury sulfate), Zhen Zha (pearls), and Hu Po (amber). All these are crushed into powders and pills rather than mixed into decoctions.

Alternatively, plant remedies are used to calm the spirit by nourishing the heart, rather than weighing down Shen. They are mainly used for palpitations, anxiety, and insomnia caused by deficient heart blood unsettling the spirit. They are also calming for deficient liver yin, which can also have a disturbing effect on the spirit.

Remedies in this category include Suan Zao Ren (wild date), Bai Zi Ren (tree of life seeds), Yuan Zhi (*Polygala tenuifolia*), Ye Jiao Teng (*Polygonum M. caulis*), and He Huan Pi (mimosa bark). The latter's Chinese name translates rather delightfully as "common happiness bark."

More Information

For more information see: **Bai Zi Ren**, page 211; **He Shou Wu**, page 114; **Suan Zao Ren**, page 210; **fundamental substances**, pages 100–101; **heart**, pages 108–109; **liver**, pages 116–117.

SUAN ZAO REN Wild date

Suan Zao Ren translates as "sour date seed" and the herb has been used in TCM since the fifth century. This herb first appeared in *Lei Gong Pao Zhi Lun* (*Grandfather Lei's Discussion of Herbal Preparations*) written around 470AD by Lei Xiao. The herb is one of the more important remedies to calm the spirit so is used for anxiety, palpitations, and insomnia, all associated with heart deficiency.

At A Glance

BOTANICAL NAME
Ziziphus jujuba var. spinosa

COMMON NAME
Wild date

FAMILY
Rhamnaceae

PART USED
Seeds

TASTE
Sweet, sour

CHARACTER
Neutral

MERIDIANS
Liver, heart

ACTIONS
Sedative, hypnotic, analgesic, lowers blood pressure, lowers body temperature

TRADITIONAL USES
• nourishes the heart and liver and calms the spirit
• prevents abnormal sweating

TYPICAL CHINESE DOSE
⅓–⅗ ounce (9–18 grams)

COMBINATIONS
Used with Fu Ling (tuckahoe), Chuan Xiong (Sichuan lovage), Zhi Mu (*Anemarrhena aspheloides*), and Gan Cao (licorice root) in Suan Zao Ren (wild date) Tang to nourish liver blood for insomnia and nervous exhaustion. Bai Zi Ren (tree of life seeds) and Wu Wei Zi (schisandra) are added for night sweats associated with kidney weakness.

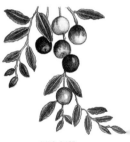

WILD DATE

Cautions

Avoid in pathogenic fire syndromes and severe diarrhea.

210

BAI ZI REN Tree of life

Twigs from the Western variety of the "tree of life" (*Thuja occidentalis*) are mainly used today as a remedy for warts, fungal skin problems, and urinary problems, although earlier generations valued the herb as a remedy for smallpox. In contrast, the Chinese species is regarded more as a sedative and has been used since the Tang Dynasty (618–907AD) as a remedy for deficient heart blood.

At A Glance

BOTANICAL NAME
Thuja orientalis

COMMON NAME
Tree of life seeds, arbor-vitae seeds

FAMILY
Cupressaceae

PART USED
Seeds

TASTE
Sweet

CHARACTER
Neutral

MERIDIANS
Heart, liver, kidney, large intestine

ACTIONS
Sedative, laxative

TRADITIONAL USES
• to nourish the heart and calm the spirit
• to moisten the intestines

TYPICAL CHINESE DOSE
⅓ ⅔ ounce (9–18 grams)

COMBINATIONS
Used with Huo Ma Ren (cannabis seeds) and Hu Tao Ren (walnuts) for constipation associated with energy weakness in the elderly or after childbirth; with Suan Zao Ren (wild date, see left) and other herbs for palpitations, insomnia, and anxiety associated with deficient heart blood; and with Wu Wei Zi (schisandra) and Mu Li (oyster shells) for night sweats caused by deficient yin.

TREE OF LIFE

Cautions

Avoid in phlegm syndromes or in cases of diarrhea.

SECRETS OF CHINESE HERBAL MEDICINE

The Soul

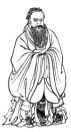

Confucius

The Chinese concept of a five-phase soul goes back to the Taoists when philosophers such as Lao Tse, and later Confucius, were active.

The soul (Ling) is a complex concept that combines aspects of energy, spiritual characteristics, and mental awareness. As with organs and body fluids, the soul falls into a pattern of five, each associated with the elements and their relevant Zang (solid) organs.

Yi

Yi, usually translated as thought, is linked to the spleen and the earth element. It is the more solid aspect of soul, implying the consciousness of possibilities and beliefs. Yi is also associated with changing those possibilities and an awareness that we can make the necessary changes. Spleen weakness can be characterized by an inability to see the possibility of change.

Hun

Hun is an ethereal aspect of soul that is difficult to translate. It resides in the liver and is linked to the wood element. It is associated with the virtues of compassion and benevolence that were highly regarded in Confucian culture. Hun is that part of the human being that survives death and it lives on for three generations. After three generations descendants stop remembering the individual by name and their Hun merges with the clan ancestors and general goodness of the world.

Zhi

Zhi is translated as will or knowing. It resides in the kidney and is linked to the water element. Zhi is associated with the Taoist views of longevity and wisdom. At birth we have plenty of congenital Jing and very little wisdom. This Jing gradually changes into wisdom so at the end of a well-lived life, with strong Zhi, there is no congenital Jing left but plenty of wisdom instead.

Shen

Shen is translated as spirit and linked with the heart and the fire element. It is not quite the same as Shen, the fundamental substance that also resides in the heart. It is described by some as a rather unspiritual concept linked more to communication and correctness.

Po

Po, the corporeal or animal soul, is associated with the lungs, so is linked to metal. It is a more physical aspect of soul than Hun and is closely associated with the seven emotions.

More Information

For more information see **five element model**, page 38; **heart**, pages 108–109; **kidney**, pages 204–205; **liver**, pages 192–193; **lungs**, pages 192–193; **spleen**, pages 116–117.

GLOSSARY

Allopathy Western medical treatment

Angina pectoris Heart pains caused by a restricted blood flow due to hardening of the coronary arteries.

Asthma Spasm of the bronchi in the lungs, narrowing the airways.

Bi syndrome Literally "pain syndrome"—a term usually applied to arthritis-like conditions.

Bronchitis Inflammation of the bronchi, the tubes that take air to the lungs.

Channels Invisible pathways in which Qi travels; also called meridians. They appear in and on the body.

Damp In Chinese medicine, damp is considered to be a yin pathogenic influence, leading to sluggishness, tired and heavy limbs, and general lethargy.

Decoction An herbal preparation, in which the plant material has been boiled in water and reduced to make a concentrated extract.

Deficient condition One where there is a lack of basic constituents (i.e. Qi, blood, or body fluids) or where there is an inadequate function of any Zang-Fu organ.

Edema A painless swelling caused by fluid retention.

Eight Principle patterns The system of organizing diagnostic information in Chinese medicine according to the principles of yin, yang; interior, exterior; hot, cold; excess, deficiency.

Excess condition One where there is a surplus or congestion of basic constituents (i.e. Qi, blood, or body fluids) or where there is inadequate function of any Zang-Fu organ.

External In Chinese medicine, any factors that influence the body from outside.

Five elements The system in Chinese medicine based on observations of the natural world. The system is built around the elements of water, wood, fire, metal, and earth.

Fu The hollow yang organs of the body.

Hypertension Describes raised blood pressure.

Internal In Chinese medicine, it refers to aspects of disharmonies that arise within the body.

Jin-Ye (body fluids) Jin refers to the lighter fluids, Ye to the denser fluids.

Jing The vital essence that is the source of life and individual development.

Marrow In Chinese medicine it is seen as the substance that makes up the brain and spinal column.

Materia medica
Substances used in medicine; the science of their properties and use.

Meridians The channels through which vital energy flows in the body. In Chinese acupuncture, there are 59 meridians in all (12 main ones).

Phlegm In Chinese medicine, disharmony of the body fluids produces either external (visible) phlegm, or internal (invisible) phlegm.

Qi The Chinese term for the life force or vital energy of the universe, which is fundamental to all aspects of life. It permeates the whole body and is concentrated in the channels.

QiGong A series of exercises associated with the breath.

San Jiao Or Triple Burner, controls the distribution of heat and fluids around the body.

Shen Spirit, a fundamental substance and expression of the life force; one of the "three treasures" of Chinese medicine, seen in the brightness of the eyes.

Ta'i-chi A form of exercise and meditational practice commonly associated in the West with martial arts.

Tang Soup A traditional decoction and method of taking herbs.

Tao/Taoism Chinese philosophical and spiritual system. Tao literally means "the way."

Three treasures The collective term that is used to describe Qi, Jing, and Shen.

Tincture An herbal remedy prepared in an alcohol base.

Tonification A process in Chinese medicine that involves strengthening the blood and Qi.

Wei Qi Defensive Qi, which protects the body from invasion by external pathogenic factors. It flows just beneath the skin.

Xue The Chinese term for blood.

Yang One aspect of the complementary opposites in Chinese philosophy. Reflects the more active, moving, warmer aspects; *see also* yin.

Yin One aspect of the complementary opposites in Chinese philosophy. Reflects the more passive, reflective, cooler aspects; *see also* yang.

Zang The solid yin organs of the body.

Zang-Fu The term used in traditional Chinese medicine for the complete yin and yang organs of the body (different from those of Western anatomy).

Exploring TCM Further

How to find a practitioner

Although there are TCM practitioners working from herbal retail outlets in most large towns and cities, qualifications and experience vary. In some cases conventionally trained orthodox health-care professionals from the Far East have found it more profitable to establish TCM clinics rather than enter established Western health services and their TCM training can be limited. Always check a reliable register of qualified practitioners before using herbalists. Many Western-trained herbalists have also undertaken additional TCM training or can advise on reputable TCM alternatives.

Buying Chinese herbs

The quality of herbs imported from China varies enormously and in many cases the labels bear little relation to the products on offer. Buying from Chinatown can be hazardous because it is difficult for non-Mandarin speakers to pronounce Chinese names convincingly. Also, many herbal outlets are run by Hong Kong Chinese who speak Cantonese rather than Mandarin so they often use different names for the herbs. There are several Western companies now importing Chinese herbs and herb products, and these will often employ a Chinese pharmacist to authenticate material. Wherever possible buy herbs pre-packaged by companies in the US, Singapore, Japan, or Europe rather than those marketed by companies in mainland China, which are often of doubtful authenticity. Some Western importers also offer mail-order services.

Useful Addresses and Further Reading

Useful Addresses

American Association of Oriental Medicine
433 Front Street
Catasauqua PA 18032
Tel: (610) 266-1433
Fax: (610) 264-2768
www.aaom.org

American Herblists Guild
1931 Gaddis Road
Canton, GA 30115
Tel: (770) 751-6021
Fax: (770) 751-7472
www.healthy.net/herbalists

The Herb Society of America
9019 Kirtland
Chardon Road
Kirtland, OH 44094
Tel: (440) 256-0514
Fax: (440) 256-0541
www.herbsociety.org

National Acupuncture and Oriental Medicine Alliance
14637 Starr Road
Southeast Olalla
WA 98359
Voice: 253-851-6896
Fax: 253-851-6886
www.actuall.org/index.html

Further Reading

BEINFIELD, H., and KORNGOLD, E., *Between Heaven and Earth,* Ballantine Books, 1991

BENSKY, D., and GAMBLE, A., *Chinese Herbal Medicine,* Eastland Press, 1982

FOSTER, S., and YUE, C., *Herbal Emissaries,* Healing Arts Press, 1992

HOBBS, C., *Medicinal Mushrooms,* Botanica Press, 1995

HOLMES, P., *The Energetics of Western Herbs,* Artemis Press, 1989

KAPTCHUK, T., *Chinese Medicine: The Web that has no Weaver,* Rider, 1983

LIU, Y.-C., *The Essential Book of Traditional Chinese Medicine,* Columbia University Press, 1988

ODY, P., *Practical Chinese Medicine,* Godsfield Press, 2000

ODY, P., LYON, A., and VILNIAC, D., *The Chinese Herbal Cookbook,* Kyle Cathie, 2000

YANG, S.-Z. trans., *The Divine Farmer's Materia Medica,* Blue Poppy Press, 1998

YEUNG, H.-C., *Handbook of Chinese Herbs and Formulas,* Institute of Chinese Medicine, 1985

INDEX

ACKNOWLEDGMENTS

PICTURE ACKNOWLEDGMENTS

Every effort has been made to trace copyright
holders and obtain permission.
The publishers apologize for any omissions and
would be pleased to make any
necessary changes at subsequent printings.

The Bridgeman Art Library, London
18T, Downe House.

Corbis, London
18B, Karen Tweedy-Holmes; 19T, Martin B
Withers; 21T, Eric and David Hoskings; 22B,
Phil Schemeister; 61, Karen Su.

Images Colour Library, London
30, 168.